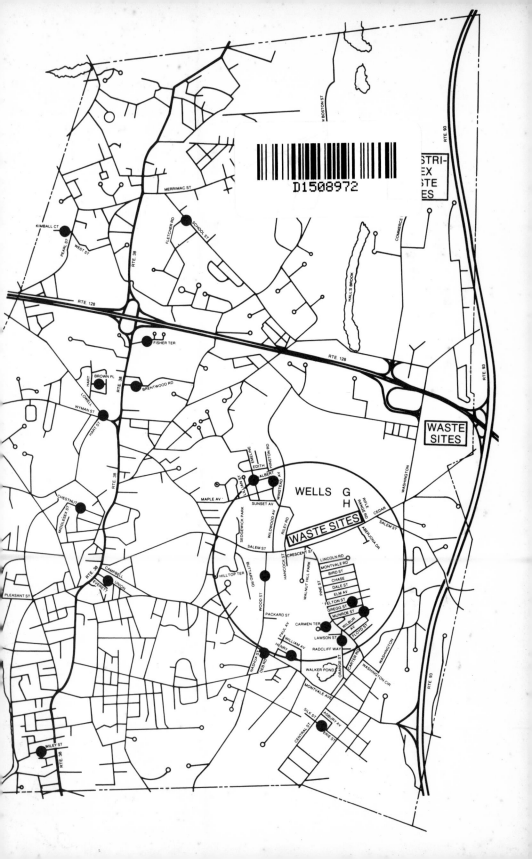

CLUSTER MYSTERY

CLUSTER MYSTERY

Epidemic and the Children of WOBURN, Mass.

Paula DiPerna

THE C. V. MOSBY COMPANY

ST. LOUIS • NEW YORK • TORONTO

For information contact The C.V. Mosby Company, 11830 Westline Industrial Drive, St. Louis, Missouri 63146

Printed in the United States of America

Library of Congress Cataloging in Publication Data

DiPerna, Paula.
  Cluster mystery.

  Includes index.
    1. Leukemia in children—Massachusetts—Woburn.
  2. Hazardous wastes—Environmental aspects—Massachusetts
  —Woburn. I. Title.
  RJ416.L4D56   1985   614.5′999   85-13788
  ISBN 0-8016-1301-9

GW/D/D 9 8 7 6 5 4 3 2 1   03/B/382

To Jimmy Anderson,
who could not know what significance was bred
by his short and special life

Contents

Acknowledgments

Now and then a writer is fortunate enough to come upon a story whose relevance seems unusually close. The events in Woburn, Massachusetts—in their implications for public policy and basic science research and their message about the importance of the individual in resisting mediocrity in leadership—seemed to sound a theme of particular importance in our age. Too, the courage with which the children at the heart of the story fought their disease is a reminder of what moral strength and human integrity really mean. That their ordeals may have been visited upon them by the contamination of natural resources surely is a matter not easily put aside.

There are people too numerous to mention who helped me in this project. Persons involved in public agencies of record trusted me to render accurately the letter and spirit of what they said. Many busy people gave me time and important aid in understanding this or that technicality. I am grateful for the extra care such people enabled me to try to take.

I want to thank especially Robert W. Stock of *The New York Times Magazine*, Jane Wilson, and Sherry Huber for recognizing all the elements at work in the chronicle, and Dr. John Truman for a thoughtful talk on the nature of medicine. The Fund for Investigative Journalism provided important support. But mostly I must thank the families involved who shared not only facts but feelings with me.

I would like to specifically mention Bruce Young, who, though long at the center of the events, retains a compelling modesty, and Donna Robbins, Kevin Robbins, the Kane family, in particular Kevin Kane, Jr., Mary and Richard Toomey, Pat and Joan Zona, Roland and Kathryn Gamache, and others who shared their personal thoughts on difficult subjects.

I would like to especially thank Charles Anderson, Jr., and Christine Anderson, who gave up a good deal of privacy so that I might tell the story of their family. And, of course, Anne Anderson, whose grace, intelligence, and patience, as well as her unwavering belief that all one needs in order to find the truth is the will to look, were inspirations for this book. Without her cooperation it could not have been written.

Paula DiPerna

1

A New Epidemic

THE PUMPING STATIONS of wells G and H in East Woburn, Massachusetts, stand abandoned, their wiring rusting in the rain that freely falls through their decaying roofs. The brushy fields outside are strewn with blackened pipe pieces, and uncoiled pipe casings lay like great slashed snakes. The wells, out of use and yet a source of talk, once carried water up from under the earth into the modest homes of Woburn.

On June 24, 1975, the Massachusetts Department of Health wrote a letter about the wells to the Board of Water Commissioners at Woburn addressed to no individual by name. The letter was a formal reply to a request from the town of Woburn to change the chlorination system of wells G and H. The department approved the change from Calgosil to Calgon-TG 10. But in the same breath the department also recommended that the town not rely on these wells because of the poor quality of their water, namely, the high concentrations of minerals and salts that caused bad taste and foul odor. The department in fact urged the town to either treat the well water to make it more acceptable or find other sources of supply. While the town gave thought to how it could comply, the wells supplied an increasing

1

amount of water to meet the demands of the growing industrial suburb 11 miles north of Boston.

In the summer of 1975 the Anderson family of East Woburn—Anne, her husband, Charles, and their children, Christine, Charles, Jr., and Jimmy—put on stiff, shiny bright yellow slickers when they, along with other tourists, faced the cool, blue-white mist of Niagara Falls. They were vacationing for the first time in years. Then the family drove on to Ohio to visit friends. They planned a trip to King's Island, where life-size Hanna-Barbera cartoon characters like Fred and Wilma Flintstone walked among delighted crowds. Jimmy Anderson was just seven then, but when one of the children in the family the Andersons were visiting felt too sick to make the King's Island outing, it was Jimmy, small for his age with thin, sandy blonde hair, who best understood.

Jimmy had just completed three and a half years of intensive treatment for acute lymphocytic leukemia, a malignancy of the lymphocytes, a type of white blood cell. Weakened from radiation and massive doses of strong chemotherapy, his daily activities had been hinged to when he was scheduled for a treatment and how well he felt afterward. Jimmy had lived most of his life thus far as a spectator, looking on at the events other children took for granted as he battled the odds to stay alive.

But this summer, in Ohio, illness was behind him, and because he felt better, he simply suggested to his parents and their friends that they wait until the other child felt better too. They did, and once at King's Island, Jimmy had great fun, even riding the roller coaster, laughing in easy confidence both with and at his mother when she shrieked in fear at the careening path of the ride. For practically the first time since infancy, Jimmy Anderson was filling up with the pleasure and excitement of life.

That spring he had contracted chicken pox, despite the best efforts of his parents to isolate him from his brother who had already caught the disease. Jimmy's body became covered with pock marks, which his mother was instructed to count every day—first, Jimmy's head, then torso, then each arm, each leg. She counted every single pock, then phoned the numbers in to Jimmy's physician who was monitoring closely to see if or how fast the disease was accelerating, for what is an ordinary infection in a normal child can run a deadly course in a child with leukemia whose infection-fighting white blood cells are not functioning normally.

Jimmy was hospitalized in the intensive care unit at Massachusetts General Hospital, critically ill with the feverish side effects, including pneumonia, of his bout with chicken pox. His mouth, eyes, even his rectum were swollen with spots. His body was so covered with the disease his mother could find only one clear, unpocked spot on his scalp to caress without discomforting him, and she gently rubbed it with her index finger while she spoke soft words to his closed eyes. Jimmy recovered.

As if to celebrate, and expecting to no longer have the high medical bills associated with Jimmy's leukemia treatment, that summer the Anderson family took their vacation and also bought a small wooden cottage at Epping, New Hampshire, set in the deep woods of a campground operated by the Methodist church. They moved in right after the Ohio trip to spend the rest of the summer, and that fall they joined thousands of other Americans anticipating the bicentennial of the United States and took a tour of the Freedom Trail. Jimmy's parents walked tranquilly over the historic Minuteman Bridge at Concord, Massachusetts, while Jimmy skipped ahead. His mother, a tall, blonde woman with smoky blue-gray eyes lush with feeling for her son, watched him almost disbelievingly, for she had never seen Jimmy with so much energy before.

Once back in Woburn, she happily signed him up for the hockey lessons he had been eager to take in order to keep pace with his athletic older brother, Chuck. But a few days later, despite Niagara Falls and King's Island and Epping and the Lexington-Concord Bridge, Anne Anderson had to ask for the hockey lesson deposit money back. The remission of Jimmy's leukemia, and with it the illusion of Jimmy's health, had shattered. On September 15, Jimmy's routine blood monitoring tests showed that the rapacious leukemia cells had returned to his system. So buoyed had she been by what had seemed like a real remission and confident that the disease was gone, Jimmy's mother had not even noticed that his body was again showing telltale bruises related to blood system clotting dysfunction. Because his doctor had to gauge how virulent a relapse had occurred, Jimmy had a painful bone marrow screening test every week through November and December. He and his family, primarily his mother, were back to the unrelenting routine of fighting his leukemia.

Jimmy Anderson was one of a group of twelve children in East Woburn who were diagnosed with leukemia, mostly of the acute lymphocytic type, between 1968 and 1979. Six of the children lived so close to each other, it would not take more than ten minutes to circle their homes in a regular, paced walk. The odds that six cases of childhood leukemia would occur within a half-mile radius by chance alone has been calculated to be a hundred to one.

The unusual number of leukemias is called a "cluster," a strange clumping of diagnoses or deaths grouped in time or place or both. A certain number of leukemias, of course, is expected in any given population. A certain number is normal. If this normalcy were plotted on graph paper, a cluster would appear as a jagged peak in an otherwise straight line. And if several unusual clusters were plotted on graph paper as a series of pointy peaks, the Woburn cluster would look like a Swiss Alp in relation to the rest, for the Woburn disease pattern was very very unusual. According to the National Cancer Institute, the average incidence of leukemia, which has no known cause, is 3.74 cases per 100,000 children. In Woburn, a town of 36,000, between 1979 and 1985 twenty-six cases were diagnosed, mostly in East Woburn. Of these, fifteen children had died by the summer of 1985.

Not only are there childhood leukemias in Woburn, but other cancers and other diseases as well. In fact, where two rambling, wooded streets without sidewalks meet in East Woburn, an adult with chronic myelocytic leukemia, a different leukemia type, lives across the street from another adult who died of lymphoma, a malignancy of the lymph nodes that produces white blood cells, who lives diagonally opposite the home where one of the original twelve children lived until his death in 1974, within sight of a home of another of the children who died in 1980. It is a remarkable intersection of cancer. There are other notable circumstances in Woburn as well.

On May 22, 1979, wells G and H, which served Jimmy Anderson's home and most other East Woburn residences, were ordered closed immediately by the State of Massachusetts' environmental protection agency, the Department of Environmental Quality Engineering (DEQE). Quite apart from the minerals and salts discussed in 1975, the water was found to be contaminated with high concentrations of chemicals shown to have been cancer-causing in laboratory animals, including chloroform, perchloroethylene (PCE), trichloroethane, and trichloroethylene (TCE). Then on September 10, 1979, news broke in the *Woburn Daily Times and Chronicle* that 300 acres of toxic chemical wastes had been unearthed the previous June in Woburn but not reported to the public. The dump included subterranean pools of arsenic and chromium and other substances, and the site was eventually designated one of the ten most hazardous in the United States. Into 1985, toxic waste sites and information about poor past waste disposal practices were still coming to light in Woburn.

There was no question that there could have been a link between the extensive toxic waste dumping, the contamination of wells G and H, Jimmy Anderson's leukemia, and the leukemias of all the other children. The question was how to find out.

Charles and Anne Anderson were married in Boston in 1961, and they moved to East Woburn in 1965. The ranch-style house they bought on Orange Street had been built in the late 1950s. They liked it well enough but chose it chiefly for one reason—its master bedroom was the first they had seen that could accommodate all the furniture in their oversize walnut bedroom set. Anne Anderson, then twenty-eight years old, telephoned her best friend, Carol Gray, who already lived in Woburn, excited about the prospect of moving to the town. East Woburn had a rural quality, lent it by tall, shady trees, the apparently pristine Walker Pond, and the general feeling of open space despite the relative proximity of the houses. The Andersons looked forward to living only 11 miles from Boston, a few blocks from their friends, the Grays, and filling out their family in what seemed an ideal setting.

The ruralness the Andersons sensed in the 1960s clung to the fringes of Woburn, which had been expanding ever outward since its founding in the seventeenth century. The district of "Wobourne" was incorporated in 1642 in an area the Indians had called *Mishawum*, or "little neck." The town had been settled by English gentlemen with the idea that they would clear a farmers' community from what the historian Samuel Lewall called "unredeemingly wild forest," plentiful with fur-bearing animals, including otter.

In 1700 taxes in Woburn were paid by 187 people, and by 1725 this tax base had increased to 305. By the time of the American Revolution the population had swelled to 1,691 people. But by the 1850s the principal business of Woburn had changed from agriculture to leather. Indeed, in 1865, of 241 children born in Woburn, 138 were born to families whose fathers worked in the many Woburn tanneries.

Supported by the tannery income, and later by a

large chemical industry, Woburn continued to increase in size, and its woods and rutted paths were replaced by paved roads carrying more people. Woburn became a full-scale Boston suburb.

Today's Woburn, with a population of approximately 36,000, is an architectural tumble of styles that have come and gone. There is a section called "the estates," an older neighborhood where elaborate gracious buildings suggest the main houses of turn-of-the-century lake resorts with oval, white and red marbled glass insets that look more like opals than windows in the walls. The streets are hilly, and tall pine trees here and there shade the full wraparound porches and lend the homes a sense of country isolation.

West Woburn has its nexus at Four Corners, a nondescript traffic circle where the boxy bank building looks the same as the 7–11 store, which, save for the arches, might as well be a McDonald's, which has a lot in common with the Fotomat. Four Corners joins this mercantile sameness along newly widened roads that pass the city hall and eventually narrow again into Main Street.

Here a few old storefronts, like Gorin's with its crushed-purple, mirrored glass, retain an art deco look and have yet to give way to quick-brick and aluminum façades. Main Street meets small business needs— Xerox, donuts, hardware, even lunch with a sense of humor at a delicatessen that serves a "Lana Tuna" sandwich, or a "Ham It Up" accompanied by a side order of "There Oughta Be a Slaw."

At The Donut Shoppe, early morning sees a gathering of locals at the counter who drink coffee and chat on about what is happening around town. The bulletin board above the counter carries posters and bits of paper announcing community events, and one main message: "you grow up the day you have the first real laugh at yourself."

This coziness, however, soon melts away into the 800 acres of northeast Woburn known as Industri-Plex Industrial Park. The two motels positioned at the entrance offer only a view of highways, long, low steel warehouses, and brown brick office buildings with such narrow, slitted windows they seem to be squinting in the sun.

Industri-Plex is not a manufacturing center but rather a distribution and repair base for a number of different industries. China, furniture, lamps, digital equipment, and other goods travel in heavy trailer trucks from Industri-Plex warehouses to retail establishments throughout New England. Or, for example, if a toaster's wires burn out, there is a good chance it would be sent to Industri-Plex for warranty replacement.

Oddly, here too a putrid, acrid smell comes and goes, twinging the nose. Known locally as the Woburn odor, it can penetrate an auto with tightly closed windows. The odor emanates from mounds of rotting, chemical-soaked hides left over from the days of Woburn's greatness as a tannery center. The hides were uncovered during the construction of Industri-Plex, but despite the smell, 21,000 people spend their work days at Industri-Plex. At each intersection in the complex, hanging, wooden, slatted signs like those at sprawling resorts pointing the way to the tennis courts and beach point the way to Digital and Diebold and Bausch and Lomb.

Picnic tables are scattered around the sparse grass, and people seem to use them, occasionally leaving litter behind.

Shiny, bright red, yellow, and green bulldozers and cranes provide the only color in this otherwise colorless panorama. The gleaming machines shove black earth into piles to be pushed into already blackened water, making new land for the still-expanding industrial park.

The Industri-Plex site is bordered by wetlands, lands geologically categorized as having a layer of fresh water just below the surface. Wetlands range from outright swamp, like the Everglades, to weedy fields that are not wet until digging liberates the hidden water. Most of the land at Industri-Plex is of the latter type—its surface looking as crumbly and dry as an old saltine.

But unfortunately at Industri-Plex it is not just water that lies below. Off behind a Cyclone fence white streamers flutter from pipe test wells sunk into the ground. Signs order "Keep Out—Danger," for within sight and smell of the offices and warehouses of Industri-Plex businesses is the 300-acre tract of toxic wastes, including the once subterranean lagoons of chromium, arsenic, and lead. The pools had languished undiscovered for decades until Charles Ryan of the *Woburn Daily Times* broke his story in September 1979. It was this discovery that earned Woburn a place on the "top ten" list of most dangerous waste sites in the United States.

According to the federal Environmental Protection Agency, there are approximately 22,000 of these sites known in the United States to date, and millions of Americans live near them. Whether sunken in lagoons, abandoned in rotting barrels, or left straight on the earth, toxic wastes can waft into the air or seep into the underground water supplies on which half the population of the United States depends for drinking.

The toxic waste issue has come to the fore only since the summer of 1978—when reporter Michael Brown, then of the *Niagara Gazette*, began to break the story that the Hooker Chemical Company had been dumping toxic materials over a period of many years into the Love Canal area near Buffalo, New York, without the knowledge of residents or town officials. Unusual patterns of birth defects and other diseases were seen among those who lived close to the canal.

Toxic wastes present two types of problems: immediate and future. Immediately, toxic materials are a dangerous, often lethal, impurity introduced to a given environment, somewhat like having raw lye lying around in a pool under one's sink. It is toxic in itself, and common sense dictates one should remove the lye before an accident occurs. A child or a pet, for example, might wander along and play with the lye and get burned. On the other hand, conceivably one could leave the lye there forever and never suffer ill-effects from it, provided one had no contact with it.

The future effects of not removing the lye are unknown, and so are the future effects of toxic waste sites. We know that if one were to take a swim in the toxic lagoons at Woburn, one would get very sick and probably die. Arsenic, for example, can kill instantly, being a favorite poison in dramas and spy thrillers. But the chronic effects of acutely poisonous substances, like arsenic, are not understood by today's medical science. We do not know how these substances behave over the long term, when human contact with them is indirect. Does a Cyclone fence, for example, sufficiently separate human beings from the problem? How are wastes transported as airborne pollution? How do they migrate through the layers of the earth into underground water? Are they already resident in human bodies, any one human body, and if so, since when? How can we possibly know, since toxic wastes are, for the most part, invisible and silent?

It would seem logical that a substance deemed toxic, that is, by definition dangerous to life —from the Greek *toxikon*, meaning a poison into which arrows are dipped—would harm human health. But exactly how substances known to be potentially hazardous to health actually do harm is one of the great medical issues of our time. It is in essence the question of how a potential threat becomes real.

Unfortunately, when environmental hazards, in particular carcinogens, those substances that can cause cancer, do affect human health, they often give no warning of their presence. There is no presymptom message that says, "I am about to give you a headache or a skin rash or a tumor." And cancer-causing substances not only give no warning, they can produce the disease as long as forty years after the body was exposed to the carcinogen. A 1986 cancer may have had its inception in 1946. Maybe, and maybe not.

With all these unsettled medical and scientific questions in the field of environmental health, those searching for cause-and-effect relationships are out of luck, for an oozing drum does not neatly equate to a smoking gun. Yet all around America there are signs that the presence of toxic wastes could be having health effects in the form of clusters of disease like Woburn's, for in many clusters, by definition unusual events, the only other unusual circumstance is often the presence or proximity of a toxic waste site or other environmental anomaly. But still, one cannot say definitely that the cluster was caused by environmental contamination. One cannot even say for sure that the cluster is "associated" with the presence of contamination in general or toxic wastes in particular.

Association is a preferred word of epidemiology, the science of causes of disease, and though it seems to be a synonym for *link*, it is not. For example, love is associated with romance, but not necessarily linked to it. One can occur without the other. The same is true in medical matters, and how an association grows into a link, if it does, is really a matter of degree. How often romance leads to love or vice versa determines the strength of the association. How unfailingly does one follow the other?

Most physicians now feel enough research has been completed to support a firm association between smoking and lung cancer. If a patient is diagnosed with the latter, most physicians will automatically ask about the former. Yet still a debate rages in some quarters as to whether there is an irrefutable cause-and-effect relationship. Certainly the tobacco industry denies the link, and certainly many Americans continue to smoke. And cigarettes are a specific, easily visible "cause."

When the potential causes of a disease are diffuse, dispersed over miles of space and years of time, forging links from associations becomes a complicated business.

As Dr. Glyn C. Caldwell, formerly of the federal Centers for Disease Control in Atlanta, a veteran of two decades of cluster study, puts it, "When everybody gets sick after eating the Sunday night tuna fish dinner, you can check the dinner. But when it comes to environmental agents, there is a whole menu of potential hazards to check." And the meal or meals may have been ingested years prior to illness.

There are scientists who believe that public concern over health effects of toxic substances and environmental pollution is exaggerated and misplaced. There are others who believe in toxic time bombs and that the clusters we see are an early visible fraction of a large health problem and that we, that is, the industrialized world, are living through what might be termed a new epidemic. The debate is lively, often heated and bitter, and it has not only medical implications but economic, political, and social ones as well.

As we struggle to determine if we are facing a new epidemic, what seems at minimum clear is that to confront it, we would need a new brand of epidemiology. Environmental detectives are like the physicians and surgeons at the turn of the century hot on the heels of the cause of malaria, except the diseases are multiple and the mosquitoes are many. Traditional ideas of cause and effect and what constitutes proof, particularly legal proof, are challenged by the sheer complexity of the causes and the effects. And into this drift every now and then a cluster of disease, like the leukemias in Woburn, pops up to demonstrate how little we know.

Clusters tug at the national sleeve, pointing out the huge hollow between scientific knowledge and the national need to protect public health and control environmental contamination. Contemporary science cannot even tell us whether a cluster is just a freak of coincidence, whether a group of cancers ten times the national average in number is just a matter of bad luck.

A cluster poses basic unanswered scientific questions, baring the heart of what remains to be known about how harmful substances in the environment actually undermine human health, causing disease in general and cancer in particular.

In particular, in the case of Jimmy Anderson, could a toxic chemical or chemicals in the water reaching his home have sent one normal white cell in his blood on a mad reproductive journey to become deadly, greedy leukemia cells that only potent chemotherapy can keep at bay?

The leukemia cluster in Woburn was eventually translated to a map that Anne Anderson and others compiled. Blue pushpins indicate the homes of children who have died of leukemia since 1968, and red ones indicate homes of children diagnosed with the disease who are still alive. Twelve pins huddle in East Woburn, tightly grouped around the Anderson house, four blue pins so close together their plastic pinheads practically touch.

Common people, Anne Anderson and friends, fashioned the map because their common sense inferred a connection between the high leukemia incidence, the toxic waste, and the polluted G and H wells. Untrained, they nevertheless worked like epidemiologists, instinctively pursuing leads. They gathered information with little outside support and in the face of widespread official indifference. But from their small community to the chambers of the United States Congress and court-rooms around the country, the questions they raised about toxic wastes and human health now reverberate in public forums.

The problem is that science lags behind public concern. What we know is not yet up to what we may sense, although for Jimmy's community, in particular for his mother, the connection between environmental contamination in Woburn and the pattern of leukemias was as plain as geography and as inescapable as putting in another pushpin on the map. The detective work at Woburn and the keen eyes and broken hearts it involved demonstrated how unscientific heroism can sometimes give a lead to science. In this, the small boy's ordeal that was the life of Jimmy Anderson gradually became the chronicle of a town and a medical touchstone for the nation.

2

Clusters or Coincidence?

CLUSTERING is a mysterious medical phenomenon loose-
ly defined as an apparent outbreak of disease clumped
in time, place, or both. An epidemic, on the other hand,
is defined as a prevalence of a disease in a particular
area rapidly affecting a great number of people. Epidemics—their effects and their misunderstanding—
have been a force shaping history, and the signs they
have left behind can be found throughout the world.

For example, visitors to the Cathedral of Santo Domingo in the Dominican Republic, the oldest cathedral
in the New World, built in 1514, will note that the building was constructed of coral stones taken from the reefs
that surround the city. However, later when an epidemic
of fever hit the city—yellow fever as it turned out—the
citizenry of Santo Domingo believed that the coral
might be giving off some insalubrious vapor that was
causing the fever. So the porous, bubbly looking stone
was sealed over with stucco. Of course, coral had had
nothing to do with the fever, which is caused by a virus
carried by the *Aedes aegypti* mosquito.

Epidemiology is the science of the search for the
cause of an epidemic, and so it is a science of shaving
in, of coming closer and closer to an answer through

17

deduction, induction, and the process of elimination. It is a matter of following clues and perhaps, above all, asking the right questions.

The word itself derives from the Greek *epi*, meaning upon, and *demos*, meaning people. In general the epidemiological method calls for first defining the problem, then collecting all available information to reveal what knowledge is missing, followed by forming the hypothesis, testing it, and then drawing conclusions. It is an inherently logical approach with a fundamental drawback where toxic wastes and environmental hazards are concerned: to define the problem, investigators must be aware that the problem is occurring; and even if they are, evidence and clues may have slipped away, slipped the mind, before an investigation takes place. The trail, in other words, particularly of physical evidence, can easily grow cold.

Thomas Sydenham, who lived in England from 1624 to 1689, is considered the father of Western epidemiology because he championed extrapolating causes from basic clinical observations. Quantifying epidemiology began in England in the late seventeenth century when public health services observed and recorded differences in the health of urban residents compared to country residents.

But in some ways epidemiology began with Hippocrates himself in the fourth century BC. His work "Airs, Water and Places" urged a consideration of the basic elements as direct or contributing causes of disease, subject to differing climatic conditions. Air could become contaminated by decay of organic matter in the earth, for example. Until the discovery of microorganisms by Louis Pasteur in the late 1800s, aided by the perfection of the use of the microscope by Anton van Leeuwenhoek in the 1600s, the miasmatists held sway, namely those who believed disease was carried in air poisoned by decaying plants and animal matter or by unspecified other corruptions in the atmosphere. William Boghurst, an apothecary and philosopher, wrote in London in 1666 of the bubonic plague, one of the world's fastest moving diseases, "Plague of pestilence is a most subtle, peculiar, insinuating, venomous, deleterious exhalation, arising from the maturation of the Faeces of the Earth, extracted into the Aire by the heat of the sun, and difflated from place to place by the winds and most tymes gradually but some tymes immediately aggressing apt bodyes." The plague, we now know, is caused by a bacteria hosted by rodents.

There was also the notion that diseases which spread quickly, like plague and cholera, attacked people disposed to deserve their sickly fate, namely sinners and the filthy. For example, in 1849, when the United States was in the grip of a cholera epidemic, the cause of cholera being still unknown, President Zachary Taylor declared August 3 a day of fasting as a godly gesture so the nation could ward off the illness.

The concept of infection and the idea that an individual could pass along a disease with no help from decaying morality or poison vapors were still young in the mid-1800s. And indeed the history of epidemiology can be described as the story of shifting emphasis between the miasma theory, the individual disposition theory, and the contagion theory. And often, it was an either/or choice.

During the great debates, for example, over how to control cholera many physicians observed that the disease tended to clump, especially in dirty neighborhoods and tenements. But when contagionists argued their position, public health officials focused on the role of the victims in the cause, suggesting that if indeed people passed the disease along themselves through their persons, then cleaning up public facilities would be futile because the disease would flourish anyway among individuals. Indeed, merchants argued that the quarantines imposed by health authorities stifled trade and free commerce. In his book *The Cholera Years*, published by the University of Chicago Press in 1962, Dr. Charles E. Rosenberg cites a survey conducted between 1832 and 1834 of 109 physicians in the United States on the causes of cholera. Forty-eight of eighty-seven still believed it to be due to "some substance added to the atmosphere or a change in atmospheric constituents"; overall ninety believed the disease was not contagious; five believed it was primarily contagious; and in a variation on the theme, fourteen believed the cause was "contingent on contagion."

Interestingly, according to Rosenberg, though the prevailing view among the professional medical community was that cholera was not contagious, many ordinary people who lived packed in the teeming quarters of the city believed indeed that the disease passed from one victim to the next.

That cholera might be carried by water was a rather novel idea in the mid-1800s, although there was a suggestion in New York City that citizens refrain from eating oysters since this food seemed to have something to do with the disease in that some upper-class victims remembered having eaten oysters prior to developing symptoms. The lack of awareness of the role of water itself in transmitting disease stands in marked contrast to our own view, which attributes a good deal of all disease to water-borne transmission, particularly in developing nations with inadequate and unsanitary plumbing facilities.

In the nineteenth century an imaginative English anesthesiologist, John Snow, linked cholera to water-borne transmission by applying common sense to his field observations. Without having ever heard of him, Anne Anderson and others followed Snow's methods and reasoning.

In 1854 London was suffering a severe cholera epidemic. Snow had a theory that cholera was transmitted through water that carried "a deadly substance in excretus or vomitus." At the time, London was served by two different water companies, the Lambeth and the Southwark & Vauxhall, and so Snow carefully gathered statistics, which meant perusing volumes of handwritten sheets of paper about the number of cholera cases. He found more of them among those victims who drew water from the Southwark & Vauxhall. Both companies distributed their water throughout London, but the Southwark & Vauxhall drew its supplies from the lower Thames, after the river had passed through the city and picked up its raw sewage. Snow's study was a masterpiece of painstaking epidemiology for its time and is still frequently cited as a seminal example of how to test a hypothesis.

Encouraged by his results, Snow was able to resort

to even a simpler means of proof in another study. He noted an outbreak of cholera in the Broad Street area of London, and to underscore his theory about water transmission, he removed the handle on the public pump residents used to draw their water. With the pump out of commission, no water could be consumed or handled. The outbreak subsided.

Epidemiology is also a matter of following leads that may prove to be false or that peter out midway. Snow was stymied at the water and sewage per se, because without knowledge that there was a microscopic world alive around him, he could not extend his theories about water to include a microorganism in the sewage. Snow had the villain, sewage, by the collar, but until Pasteur proved the existence of microbes, he could not have the villain by the throat. It was an example of how science can be blocked by a lack of technical invention, which in turn depresses the development of theories: one piece of equipment can open a world, and the lack of equipment can keep the world sealed shut and inaccessible. In other words, Snow could only go as far as available technology would take him without risking being called a quack.

One of the greatest stories of unraveling medical mysteries surrounds the case of malaria, the symptoms of which were described by Hippocrates in ancient Greece but which were not traced to a cause until the late 1800s. Prevailing medical thought associated the disease with swampy areas early on because of their smelliness and hence the name from the Italian *malaria*, meaning bad air. However, in his fine book *Malaria and Man*, published by E. P. Dutton in 1978, Gordon Harrison states that ordinary people who lived in areas where malaria was prevalent suspected the disease was related not to the swamps but to the mosquitoes. Indeed, writes Harrison, the naturalist von Humboldt heard this theory among indigenous peoples on his Orinoco River expedition through the Amazon region of South America in the early 1800s. Harrison also quotes the French parasitologist Emile Brumpt who wrote in 1949, "If only great scientific minds had listened to the wisdom of the people, the secrets of malaria might have been exposed much sooner."

Of course, as with cholera, it was not the tiny mosquito itself but the parasite it hosted with which science had to reckon. Again, open-mindedness and technology had roles in the pace of cracking the code of the disease.

In 1878 it was known that victims of malaria had tiny black particles in their blood that at the time were believed to be residue hemoglobin in red cells. These pigments had been observed by the pathologist Achille Kelsch who found them in the blood of all living victims and noted the pigment seemed to occur when the patients were in the grip of fevers associated with the disease. Harrison notes that the "pigments" were indeed the parasites, but he also noted perceptively that the question of what the pigments were was "not his [Kelsch's] kind of question . . . pathology made him concerned with changes brought on by the disease, not the process of the disease," in the way a physician treating cancer may not be focused on learning why that cancer began but rather on arresting its progress. So Kelsch ignored the pigments and concentrated instead on the study of malaria symptoms.

Technology played its part too since Kelsch had unknowingly used a staining method on slides of blood that "froze" the pigments, that is, killed the parasites, causing them to appear immobile. But when Dr. Alphonse Laveran, a French physician with a public health interest who was working in Algeria, looked into malaria, he literally looked in a different way. He studied unstained liquid blood drops, and when he did, he saw moving, flagellating "pigments," either crescent shaped or spherical, confirming for himself that the pigments were alive. But for four years, according to Harrison, Laveran's discovery went ignored or rejected. And when Laveran went so far as to suggest the animal might be a parasite of the mosquito, he was ridiculed. Having discovered bacteria in the 1860s, thanks to Pasteur, scientists now wanted to believe all miroorganisms were bacteria.

Laveran meantime went to Italy in 1882 to see if the wiggly blood components could also be found in the blood of malaria victims there. They were. And meanwhile, unbeknownst to Laveran, Cuban doctor Carlos Finlay had begun speculating on the possible link between mosquitoes and the other dreaded tropical scourge, yellow fever.

But though this scientific cloth was being woven around the world, it was not until the time came to build the Panama Canal that there was commercial incentive enough to really get to the bottom of the mystery of tropical diseases. For with the canal project, which put workers at risk, suddenly thousands of workers were dying, and without stopping the disease, the canal could not be built. It was not until 1902, when Dr. Ronald Ross won the Nobel Prize for his work, that it was finally recognized that malaria was carried by the *Anopheles* mosquito specifically, which could inject into the body parasites that harbored the malaria virus. The canal was opened in 1914, decades after Kelsch and Laveran and the original discovery of mysterious moving particles in malarial victims' blood.

That modern epidemiologists sometimes miss a lead by ignoring and misinterpreting the instincts of laypersons is documented by Berton Roueché in his wonderful book *The Medical Detectives*, derived from his articles in *The New Yorker* magazine. Of particular interest is the tale of the Tampa man whose son had been bitten in 1953 by a bat that had been flying in strange patterns before swooping down on the boy. The father feared the possibility of rabies but was assured by a public health official that only vampire bats carried rabies; at the time the *Dasypterus floridanus* species, which had bitten the boy, was considered harmless. But the boy died, nevertheless, of rabies.

Interestingly and sadly, in 1951 a man in Texas had worriedly reported to his physician that his wife had been bitten by a bat, and he too met the prevailing view voiced by the doctor that the biting bat, also a *Dasypterus floridanus*, was "harmless." The wife too died of rabies. It took the Florida case to prompt the issuance of a public health service dispatch warning on the dangerous nature of this heretofore considered harmless species.

This is not to categorically condemn public health officials for being slow to act, for surely word takes time to travel, especially before the current age of mass media and quick information exchange. And local physicians often must count on "experts" for information, and the experts, for example, had said the bat *Dasypterus flori-danus* was harmless. But it is safe to say that scientists are both challenged by and limited by what they think they know. On the one hand, they build on previously acquired knowledge; on the other, they are hemmed in by it. What is known is secure; the unknown or yet to be proven is thin ice.

The first known case of tracing a cancer or malignancy to an environmental exposure came with the now classic work of physician Percivall Pott in London in 1775. Pott noticed that chimney sweeps particularly suffered from cancer of the scrotum, and he suggested that their diseases were related to the soot that stuck in the folds of scrotal tissue. Pott was close, but he did not realize that it was not the soot per se but the tars it contained that most likely were carcinogenic. Pott also noted that many of the ill men had been chimney sweeps as children, as young as eight or nine in some cases since the practice then was to hire young, lithe boys to slither down narrow chimneys. Pott's reasoning, based on what would in today's epidemiology be called anecdotal observation, was a precursor of the commonly accepted belief that causative environmental exposures can take place many years before the symptoms of a disease appear. This is known as the latency factor.

Pott's work stands as a landmark in the study of environmentally or occupationally induced carcinogenesis, and it was in a sense also one of the first cancer cluster investigations, for Pott's chimney sweeps, from an epidemiological point of view, represented an occupational cluster of scrotal cancer.

Perhaps the starkest cases of occupational cancer clusters came in the mid-1940s and 1950s with the appearance of a formerly rare cancer, mesothelioma, a malignancy of the lining of the lungs and stomach. Several investigators began to notice an excess of deaths from this disease, practically unheard of before, among workers suffering as well from asbestosis, a lung disease previously tied to exposure to asbestos fibers, which caused breathing difficulty as well as death.

It took many more years to establish a more-or-less irrefutable association between mesothelioma and asbestos exposure, but virtually every case of mesothelioma has been traced to an exposure to asbestos. One sad but well-known case reported by Dr. Irving Selikoff, a pioneer in the field of occupational health and asbestos research and an expert in mesothelioma, of the Mt. Sinai Hospital in New York City, involved an otherwise healthy young woman who developed the disease and whose only exposure was when, as a child, she inhaled the asbestos fibers her mother shook out of her father's clothes before washing them. Her father had been an asbestos worker.

But by the time the association between asbestos and mesothelioma was clearly established, asbestos fibers were ubiquitous in our society—lining pipes and automobile brakes, woven into cloth, and pressed into insulation tiles to make buildings safer from fire. Virtually every public school in the United States used asbestos insulation, and in August 1984, in fact, the federal government issued a report saying that about 14,000 buildings were involved and that cost of removing the asbestos would be $1.4 billion. The Johns Manville Corporation, one of the most important corporations in the asbestos industry, declared bankruptcy in August 1982 because it simply could not pay all the claims pending against it filed by workers who had suffered injury or death from asbestos exposure while they had been Manville employees.

The asbestos problem is severe and global. According to Dr. Selikoff and others, there have been 100,000 deaths due to exposure to asbestos in the United States alone, and there are estimates that even if every shred of asbestos were eliminated from use from now on, the United States would still suffer 350,000 deaths over the next ten years as a result of previous asbestos exposures.

Against these numbers a typical leukemia cluster pales in size. Leukemia is a relatively rare disease, though not rarer than mesothelioma, striking approximately 21,500 adults a year in the United States in all its forms, and 2,500 children. Leukemia is commonly referred to as cancer of the blood, and it is a malignancy that occurs in different types of white blood cells. Acute lymphocytic leukemia, Jimmy Anderson's illness, strikes when lymphocytes, a type of white cell, fail to mature to take on the infection-fighting function they are supposed to perform. Instead they run amok, wildly reproducing before they mature, snuffing out other blood cells in the way weeds can overtake healthy plants. According to Dr. John Truman, Jimmy's physician and head of pediatric oncology at Massachusetts General Hospital in Boston who has treated leukemic children for some twenty years, leukemia cells reproduce exponentially in four days, so that one leukemia cell can become a billion in a matter of three or four months if left to its own devices. The leukemia cells simply spill out of the bone marrow where blood cells are produced, like water leaking from both ends of a pipe, crowding out the normal cells. Without treatment, leukemia cells can easily add a kilogram of weight to the body, one trillion cells, and death from leukemia is in essence death from sapped energy and suffocation because the blood's red cells, which carry the body's oxygen supply, simply have no place left to go.

Treatment of leukemia therefore is a matter of attempting to kill off the renegade cells and keep them from reappearing.

What causes normal cells to become leukemic, or cancerous in any form for that matter, is not known, except scientists generally now agree that the process can occur in two stages—initiation and promotion—beginning at the level of the cell. Initiation is a kind of pump priming wherein some mechanism yet unknown programs a cell with wrong information, poising it to madly reproduce itself according to incorrect instructions. Promotion then comes along, a second mechanism akin to throwing the *on* switch to a haywire operation, that is, setting the initiated cells into motion. The promoting agent may be a carcinogenic chemical; so may be the initiating agent. In theory, in a cluster, exposure to the initiating agent, or the promoting agent, may be what the cluster victims have in common.

Leukemia clustering itself is an international phenomenon that was first scientifically described in the United States in 1937. In the mid-1950s and 1960s clusters attracted research because they presented a testable theory about the cause of leukemia—that a virus or other infectious agent could pass from one case to the next. The first major epidemiological investigation of a childhood leukemia cluster took place in Niles, Illinois, in 1963, where an increased incidence of the disease was noticed among children who seemed to have only their attendance at a particular Roman Catholic primary school in common. Their families shared no ethnic factor or occupational background. There was no common thread running through the wider community either. Levels of radiation were checked at the school and the homes of some of the children, but levels were considered to be in the "low normal" range. The search for a cause in Niles led nowhere. Between 1963 and 1983 the federal Centers for Disease Control (CDC) has conducted epidemiological investigations of 101 clusters of various types of cancer, and no cause has ever been found.

Dr. Glyn C. Caldwell, a stocky epidemiologist with a crew cut, formerly of the Chronic Diseases Division of the CDC and its Cancer Epidemiology Branch, has been involved in cluster investigations for nearly twenty years along with Dr. Clark Heath, also of the CDC. Caldwell feels comfortable enough with what he says to rock back and forth on a hardwood swivel chair as he is saying it in the offices of the CDC, a series of barrack-style buildings with rippled metal roofs behind the Internal Revenue Service in Chamblee, Georgia, outside Atlanta. He looks more like a confident auto salesman than a cautious scientist, and he puts the complexities of unraveling clusters in simple terms, patly summarizing the twin frustrations that have plagued cluster research for decades: "One, we can't tell the chance clusters from the causal ones, and among the causal ones we can't tell the causes."

In unraveling clusters, epidemiologists first study the odds. The odds are, for example, that when you flip a coin, it will land heads roughly as often as it lands tails. The odds against hitting heads ten times in a row are five to one, but it could happen. It could even happen by chance twenty or thirty times in a row. But the more times in a row heads comes up, the more suspicious one might become that the coin is weighted.

The number of times one flips the coin defines the statistical "power" of the test, roughly corresponding to the number of times the test is done, or the number of times the test needs to be done in order to observe any effect. The more times you flip and you turn up heads, the more likely the coin is weighted. Flipping ten times should make you more certain than flipping just twice.

But in leukemia clusters, because the disease is so rare, there is little statistical power in a basic statistical test. Three leukemia cases among 100 children is extremely rare and odd, odder still if the cases are all the same leukemia type. But such a clumping could be accidental—an artifact of statistics—and one cannot categorically prove it is not. In fact, according to a review of the clustering phenomenon that appeared in the standard reference book *Cancer Epidemiology and Prevention,* published in 1983, in theory even a statistically significant cluster report in the United States every week for three years in the United States might still be a chance phenomenon.

Dr. Robert C. Hoover, head of environmental epidemiology studies for the National Cancer Institute, makes the problematic point nicely: "All clusters are by definition weird events. Some are more weird than others." Weirdness then is a matter of degree.

Of course it is the weirdness that first alerts science to the presence of a cluster, and spontaneous calls from those emotionally involved are usually what first brings clusters to light. In the late 1970s and early 1980s, the CDC received roughly a call a day from people—mostly laypersons—who thought they had spotted a cluster of cancer. So in cluster epidemiology the tools of the scientist are first the telephone and note pad.

Cluster reports can be as subjective as "everyone in my neighborhood has cancer." Dr. Matthew Zack, a physician turned epidemiologist and statistician at the CDC, fields many of these calls while sitting in front of his flickering computer terminal surrounded by manila files. His work space looks more like a library than a scientific laboratory. To do his brand of statistical science, Zack must interview the callers and attempt to obtain basic blocks of information from which a cluster investigation can be built.

Cancer is not one disease but many, and different types of tumors develop in different organs, so a pure cluster from the epidemiologist's point of view is one in which the disease occurs in the same form among victims—all liver cancer, all lung cancer, for example.

Zack therefore first tries to learn what types of cancer are being reported and how many there are, addresses, age, race of the patients, and hospital, and date of diagnosis or death if possible.

Armed with this information, a cluster investigator can put the cluster report in its statistical context, the national cancer picture, which can be viewed from two angles. One is mortality, the number of cancer deaths; the other is incidence, the number of cancer diagnoses.

A cluster appears as a blip in one or both of these rates. In 1975 the National Cancer Institute published the *Atlas of Cancer Mortality*, bound volumes of tables and maps and charts that orchestrate, by county, the number of deaths from various cancer types in the United States between 1950 and 1969. It, and the United States Cancer Mortality Index, published in 1974, are the latest sources of national information on cancer deaths available. The *Atlas*, in the same tradition as geography reference books, makes information about where and how many people have died of cancer perceptible at a glance.

Incidence data are not as pat. In 1973 the National Cancer Institute began the Surveillance, Epidemiology and End Results Program (SEER). The program collects cancer diagnoses like reports of wounded from the field, extrapolating national incidence rates from a handful of states such as Iowa, Connecticut, and New Jersey plus selected urban areas such as Seattle and New Orleans. However twenty-two states now monitor themselves by requiring hospitals or physicians to report current cancer diagnoses to a centralized, often computerized state level registry. In the remaining states, however, a cancer case, unlike syphilis or tuberculosis, is not "reportable" and will slip through the data net until, and unless, it becomes a death.

The information a caller—a layperson, a public health official, an Anne Anderson perhaps—provides is then compared to what the epidemiologist would expect to see based on previous incidence and mortality data for the caller's area. How weird is the weirdness, in other words?

But approximately 90% of the callers to the CDC cannot furnish the fundamentals, and so the cluster reports are not further investigated. In the remaining 5% to 10% the CDC calculates whether what the caller has reported exceeds the rates considered to be the norm for the area in question. If there is an excess above the norm, then the cluster is considered "statistically significant" or "real." In the 90% of unpursued cluster reports, whether "real" clusters existed to prompt the report is never known.

But even a real cluster may mean no more than six or seven extra leukemia cases, not many unless these cases are you or your child. But establishing that there are indeed excess cases does not provide much information. "The problem is after the realness," comments Dr. Caldwell. "Rare events happen, however rarely."

Rareness, of course, exists only in a context, and contexts, like fashions, can change. According to Dr. Caldwell, "in the 50's and 60's we got little old ladies calling in complaining about smells from their oleander bushes. Then with the environmental movement, the calls switched to concern with chemicals and other environmental agents."

Indeed, there has been a shifting context for the cause of cancer itself, and during the reign of the oleander bush worries, many cancer scientists believed the disease was virally caused. But much research did not uncover convincing evidence for the viral theory.

Only one form of leukemia, T-cell leukemia, a malignancy of a particular type of white blood cell, has been shown to be linked to a virus. Many scientists believe that viruses may play a role in priming a cell to become cancerous, in cancer initiation, that is.

As the viral theory attracted study, society became gradually more aware of environmental pollution, and theories developed about its relationship to the development of cancer.

"With the changes in our index of suspicions about the causes of cancer in the last decades," says Dr. Joseph F. Fraumeni, Jr., chief of the Environmental Epidemiology Branch of the National Cancer Institute who grew up in Reading, Massachusetts, a stone's throw from Woburn, "our hypotheses for cancer clusters changed from viruses to chemical to other environmental agents."

Like the Percivall Pott discovery of cancer among the chimney sweeps, most investigations of environmentally caused cancers have involved occupational exposures, since in a limited workplace environment with clearly fixed and visible boundaries, clusters of disease stood out more readily than they would ambient in a city or town.

Workers in almost all jobs meet occupational hazards, but often the hazards have not been known to the workers, even if the substance in question has been shown to be hazardous in a laboratory. The first cases of asbestosis were confirmed in England in 1898, yet asbestos continued in common use. The English Parliament had even refrained from including asbestosis on a list of diseases for which the government might underwrite medical bills because, according to Dr. Selikoff, they were sure that with the discovery of the disease, asbestos use would be eliminated and the disease would eventually disappear.

Vinyl chloride, an important plastic polymer, had

been shown to be carcinogenic in laboratory animals in 1970. It nevertheless continued in wide industrial use, and in 1974 in Kentucky it was formally observed to cause cancer in humans, namely angiosarcoma, a rare form of liver cancer, among workers who handled the substance or were exposed to it.

Finding associations in the workplace has proven easier than in the open environment for obvious reasons: what comes in and out of a workplace is easier to monitor than what comes in and out and across a neighborhood. It may also be that workers are exposed to higher concentrations of particular chemicals than the rest of us are in the open environment. And indeed the occupational "model" has often been used to develop hypotheses about clusters that occur outside the workplace; for example, in unraveling clusters and searching for physical evidence, often the first substances suspected are those already shown to be dangerous. The question is how dangerous, and how much is known about how dangerous.

Benzene is a case in point. It is perhaps one of the most ubiquitous and common solvents; a can of benzene may be found under every sink in every household where old furniture has been refinished or paint has been removed. Since at least 1928 benzene has been associated with leukemia, mostly of the myelocytic type, in workers who handled the substance. Myelocytes are a granulated type of white cell, different from the ungranulated lymphocyte. And until as recently as August 1983, benzene was still generally associated mainly with myelocytic, and not lymphocytic, leukemia. But then a study of rubber industry workers by a group of epidemiologists at the University of North Carolina heightened evidence of an association with lymphocytic leukemia as well.

The example is of interest because it suggests that we may know only as much as we see, and that we may see only as much as we have yet looked for, and that though a particular chemical has not been shown to cause cancer yet, someday it may.

For now the predictor of cause is the animal test wherein mice or rats are fed a substance to see if associations appear. But this approach leads to slot machine results. For example, if a component in a household cleaner has been shown to cause liver cancer in laboratory rats, can it be blamed for skin cancer in humans? The disease is the same, but the organ and species are different. So the chemical being tested is like a coin, and the household cleaner results are like hitting cherries, oranges, and melons all across. Ironclad proof would be cherries all across: a substance known to cause liver cancer in rats is found to be the only common factor among humans in a cluster of liver cancer. But still such proof would not be irrefutable. The best we could say is there was a strong association, and therefore a likelihood that the chemical played some role in the cluster. The only "proof" of a cluster is another cluster, exactly the same diseases happening under exactly the same environmental circumstances.

Just how much cancer is caused by environmental factors, whether natural or produced by humans, is open to dispute. And all who speak of the problem do not use the word *environment* the same way. Some mean pollutants in the air and water only; others mean all things extraneous to the body itself, including diet, personal habits, and so forth. In *Malignant Neglect*, published in 1979, the Environmental Defense Fund, a leading group on the matter of public health, claimed as much as 90% of all cancer may be environmentally caused, using the word very broadly. In 1978, under the administration of President Jimmy Carter, Secretary of Health, Education and Welfare Joseph A. Califano, Jr., predicted a 20% to 30% increase in the cancer rate attributable to just six chemicals—asbestos, arsenic, benzene, chromium, nickel oxides, and petroleum fractions. The first Presidential Council on the Environment Annual Report to be published under the Reagan Administration said in 1981, "Today it is widely accepted that discrete industrial chemical substances play only a minor role in the causation of most cancers. . . . In fact, the American Medical Association's House of Delegates recently adopted a report which stated, in part, there 'is no definitive epidemiological evidence that the United States has experienced an overall increase in the incidence of cancer related to high levels of pollutants or contaminants in the environment.' "

A study by the United States Office of Technology Assessment in 1981 by two British epidemiologists, Sir Richard Doll and Richard Peto, concluded that approximately 8% of all cancers in the United States could be attributed to workplace or general environmental exposure to human-made carcinogens, accounting for 53,000 excess deaths per year.

Into this confusion of how many deaths overall can be attributed to synthetic chemical causes enters the problem of how to attribute which specific deaths and which clusters, to which causes. In environmental epidemiology the search for proof becomes a matter of

trying to arrive ever closer to the eye of the storm, looking for common factors, evaluating the probabilities of
trying to determine what chemical exposures a person
had perhaps decades before a disease appears and comparing it to what has been learned about the chemicals
in questions from laboratory data. It is a complex and
staggeringly expensive business to do such a review.
Understanding the role of asbestos has taken sixty years
and millions of dollars, and the trail of evidence was
rather uncluttered. Mesothelioma almost always led
back to asbestos.

If one must apply this constantly moving, controver-
sial, and imprecise science to the thousands of toxic
waste sites in the United States, one has a problem of
staggering proportion. For most toxic waste sites are
soups of chemicals, each containing not one potential
culprit but many. And the waste site may not be the
only source of pollution in a neighborhood. The open
environment of industrialized Buffalo itself, for example, complemented the hidden chemicals at Love Canal.
How to differentiate between the environmental agent
one breathed in the street and the one that may have
seeped up under the floor of one's basement?

And we may not see disease symptoms, especially in
cancer, until after the exposure is over. Given the latency
factor, a cancer cluster cannot be detected until many
years after it began to form. At this late date the chance
of nabbing the cause is practically nil because physical
clues will have all but disappeared. A cluster investigation, therefore, is almost predestined to be inconclusive because it is always playing catch-up to the facts
and the evidence.

That is the rudimentary state of the knowledge avail-

able in 1985. In 1972, when Jimmy Anderson was diagnosed, understanding was thirteen years less sophisticated, thirteen years cruder, thirteen years further behind. That toxic waste dumps were a nationally
significant problem was not yet suspected because their
prevalence, indeed their existence, was not yet widely
known.

3

The Early Ordeal of
Jimmy Anderson

ANNE RUSSELL ANDERSON was born on June 15, 1936, the youngest child and only daughter in a family of four children. She grew up in Somerville, a town only several miles away from Woburn. Her earliest memory, she says, is of feeling safely asway on top of the world, a toddler riding the shoulders of a favorite, very tall uncle. Her father operated a wholesale fruit business, and her mother ran the home with help from her children. Anne calculates that she may have folded 17,680 pairs of socks for her brothers and father while she was growing up.

But the Anderson household was not uninvolved in the outside world, and while Anne gained experience in homemaking rituals, she was also constantly being exposed to the lively political discussions favored by her parents. She remembers family dinners, particularly at holidays, when each child was asked his or her opinion and encouraged to express ideas about whatever was taking place in the world at the time. Anne's mother particularly had wide interests and had hoped to attend nursing school. When economics prevented her from doing so, she supplemented life with a full diet of reading. Well into her senior years, Mrs. Russell remained a thoughtful woman with deep blue eyes full of brilliant sparkle.

Anne Anderson too was inquisitive by nature. She was a bright, popular student at Somerville High School, where she had above-average grades, though she does not remember working hard to get them. During high school she gave some thought to becoming a nurse, but none of her friends were pursuing academic careers. Although Anne's brothers went off to college, Anne did not despite her mother's encouragement to do so. Instead, after graduation she took a job at the Somerville Public Library because she too loved being around books. She worked at the library for seven years, and except for clerical work she did at the Hancock Life Insurance Company during her high school senior year, the library job was her only working experience prior to and throughout her twenty-year marriage.

Anne Russell met Charles Anderson, who had grown up in East Boston, on a blind date in 1960. The two were married the next year. They spent their first years of married life with Charles Anderson completing his military service in New Jersey. Anne commuted between Massachusetts and New Jersey for weekend visits to her husband until she could join him permanently after basic training. The Andersons were often invited to parties. They loved a good time and knew how to help others have one too. Anne Anderson looks back and says, "life for us was games and laughs and fun."

But Anne felt she was born to be a mother, and indeed it gave her great personal fulfillment. The Anderson's first child, Christine, was born on November 17, 1962, and she was a beautiful, lively little girl. Somewhat demanding as an infant, she kept Anne busy full time. Charles Anderson, Jr., almost from birth nicknamed Chuckie, was born on September 13, 1966. And as Anne says, "I couldn't wait for my second to be born because I couldn't wait for that wonderful feeling of touching a newborn baby's skin. I loved that feeling, and I loved the excitement of new babies. I loved them looking at me; I loved doing things for them. I loved experiencing that special love a mother feels for a child."

Around this time, demand for water was growing in Woburn. And city officials knew that construction under way in northeast Woburn would be bringing in new businesses that would tax the water supply even further. In the early 1960s the city drew its drinking water exclusively from a series of wells in the Horn Pond area of southwest Woburn. There was no connection to the Metropolitan District Commission (MDC), a private regional water supply agency that sold water to Massachusetts communities after piping it from the Quabbin Reservoir 60 miles west of Boston.

City public works officials were aware that the Aberjona River area was rich in water. Old Woburn industries had been pumping as much as a million gallons a day through their private wells. The town therefore decided to dig two municipal wells in the Aberjona area. No surveying of the underlying geology was done, nor was there any sampling of the groundwater for other than bacteria. The sole reason for locating the wells was the promise of a plentiful water supply.

On October 1, 1964, the first of these, well G, began to pump into town mains. On July 26, 1967, well H also came on line. Primarily the wells were intended to meet warm weather extra demand in the growing Woburn suburbs, such as East Woburn.

At first, the wells provided supplementary water for only the summer months, but gradually, as demand grew, G and H remained switched on for as long as six months a year. They began providing a good deal of the water that reached the Anderson house and the houses of their neighbors. But the water quality was not good. It had a rusty kind of sour odor, as well as a strong smell of chlorine, combined with a foul, stale taste. Particles floated in it, and the linings of dishwashers and washing machines were corroded by its rushing through. Milk poured into a clean glass looked brown because the glass had become so water stained. The way other neighbors talked about the weather, East Woburn residents talked about the water, how it was each day and how it had been the day before. Anne Anderson remembers her mother used to bring over bottles of water from the family home in Somerville. "My children," says Anne with a characteristic wryness, "grew up asking not for mother's milk but for Nanna's water."

Always, though, when the residents complained to the town of Woburn, they were told the water was safe and that there was nothing wrong with it. In fact, Anne Anderson's mother grew so exasperated by the constant water problems her daughter's family had that she took a bottle of Woburn water herself to the state house in Boston and asked that it be tested. She remembers hauling in the jug and refusing to take "no" for an answer when the clerk told her that state agencies could not sample water unless requested to do so by the towns involved. Mrs. Russell coaxed, saying, "But I have the water right here?" Her attempt was unavailing. She could not get the water tested either.

Jimmy Anderson was born on July 16, 1968. He weighed 10½ pounds at birth and seemed a happy and healthy baby. Life from Jimmy's birth proceeded normally, for all intents and purposes. Charles Anderson's work as a systems analyst required a certain amount of traveling. And when he was on the road a lot, he would send back postcards to his family from exotic spots like Costa Rica. He was doing well professionally, and this period in the Anderson home, save for the complaints about the water, was marked by tranquility, family peace, and promise.

In the meantime, about 2 miles from the Anderson house, construction was moving ahead at the site of what is today Industri-Plex Industrial Park. The land had seen an overlay of owners. To take advantage of the flourishing leather business in Woburn, in 1853 an entrepreneur named Robert B. Eaton purchased a tract of land in northeast Woburn and established the Woburn Chemical Works. It produced vitriol and other caustic substances that were sold to the tanneries, as well as to the textile and paper operations that had sprung up throughout New England.

Eaton's successful business was purchased by Merrimack Chemical Company in 1863. By 1929, Merrimack had grown from 5 acres and a few buildings to 417 acres and ninety buildings. It was then one of the largest chemical manufacturers in the United States. It had also acquired the William H. Swift Company of Boston, which produced arsenic-based insecticides, the New

England Manufacturing Company, which produced TNT and other explosives, and the Cochrane Chemical Company of Everett, Massachusetts.

All the chemicals Merrimack and Eaton operations had used were either buried under or dumped on the surface of the ground.

In 1929 the Monsanto Chemical Company bought Merrimack but closed the Woburn facility in 1931, selling it to New England Chemical Company in 1934, which began producing hide and bone glue. Pig-rendering operations were begun during this period. In 1936 the facility passed to the Consolidated Chemical Industries and then to the Stauffer Chemical Company, which produced animal glue and grease on the site and acquired title in 1963 in the name of the Stauffer Chemical Company Foundation.

These operations also continued to dispose of their wastes by dumping it onto the ground or swampy lands in the area. In 1968 the property was sold to the trustees of what was called the Mark Phillip Realty Trust Company, specifically to a developer named William F. D'Annolfo. Whether D'Annolfo knew the extent of the toxic contamination of the land is not known.

In the fall of 1972 digging and thrashing began in the southern end of the site, heading north. Bulldozers thrust into buried, chemical-soaked animal hides left over from the tannery days, exposing them to the air, giving birth to the noxious, putrid smell soon to become known as the Woburn odor. Development work, however, continued.

Outside the burgeoning Industri-Plex area, there were other businesses in full swing. One, on Salem

Street, with a tall, red brick smokestack with its name inlaid in white brick was the John J. Riley Tannery, established in 1910.

On Washington Street, also a bit southeast of the Industri-Plex site, Cyrovac, Inc., a division of the W. R. Grace Company, operated a plant that produced metal packaging equipment for the food industry on land it had acquired from the Calidyne Company in 1960, which had never completed its building or done business on the property. Prior to that the property had been used for farming. Cyrovac had nearly $2 million in sales during its first year of operation.

To keep the equipment clean and free of grease or stray paint, solvents, including trichloroethylene (TCE), tetrachloroethylene, tetrachloroethane, were used at the Cyrovac factory. Over the years too, liquid waste material from the degreasing shop was disposed of by factory workers, who spread it in the stony ground behind the plant. Drums containing paint sludge that itself contained solvents were also disposed of by workers, who buried or emptied the drums in drainage pits, also located behind the plant.

In January of 1972 the weather in Woburn had been wintry and wet and all three Anderson children developed symptoms of flu—listlessness, sore throats, nausea, crankiness, and fever. Jimmy, then three and a half years old, had been particularly listless that month, and he did not recover as his brother and sister did. When he was put in his crib, he would cry for no apparent reason; both sets of grandparents saw him and said he looked unusually pale. So the Andersons took their son to see the family pediatrician who had been treating their children since birth. He took blood samples, and the Andersons took Jimmy home. It was late on Saturday afternoon when the physician phoned Anne Anderson to say he wanted to admit Jimmy to Massachusetts General Hospital for further tests.

In Anne Anderson's entire life to that point, she had known of only one child with leukemia, a distant acquaintance. She knew nothing about the disease, other than that it was potentially fatal, but she remembers that night being in the grip of the premonition that leukemia was indeed what Jimmy had and that he would be the one case she would hear of in his generation.

The Andersons had guests that weekend, and Anne tried to maintain her composure despite the tension she felt while waiting for the results. Once while preparing dinner, she began to cry and had to turn away from the other children and her family friends. Her husband, though, saw her tears and asked why she was so upset. "Because I think Jimmy has leukemia," she finally admitted. Charles Anderson attempted to allay Anne's fears, but that weekend began the inner quaking of a parent coming to terms with the prospect of the death of a child.

On the night before Jimmy was due to enter Massachusetts General, Anne Anderson could not sleep. She finally walked across the carpeted hall to Jimmy's room, unable to keep from looking at her son, and then unable to leave him. She took Jimmy into bed with her and her husband so she could watch him while he slept.

On January 31, 1972, the Andersons were told by Dr. John Truman at Massachusetts General that indeed Jimmy had acute lymphocytic leukemia. Anne Anderson's memory is of only those three words and of shafts of pure sunlight entering the room through the blinds across her back. There were a few seconds of confusion, she says, for she could not understand why, if there was so much sun in the room, she suddenly felt so cold inside.

Acute lymphocytic leukemia is a rare disease that strikes roughly 1,800 children a year in the United States. Of the childhood leukemias, it is the most common, and of the childhood cancers leukemia is the most common. Still the disease is so rare that data on incidence over several years are combined because in a single year sometimes there are not enough cases from which to extrapolate a national rate. Consequently the numbers are averaged rather than taken on a strictly annual basis. Acute lymphocytic leukemia is extremely unusual among adults, who tend to suffer from other forms of the disease. The average incidence of acute lymphocytic leukemia among children is 2.47 per 100,000 and 3.74 per 100,000 children for all types of leukemia.

The disease is potentially fatal, although it is controllable and thus curable in up to 75% of the cases treated these days, according to the American Cancer Society. In 1972 the odds of Jimmy's surviving were roughly 50% according to his physician, John Truman, who remembers the days when a diagnosis of leukemia was a certain death sentence. "My great frustration in my early days as a physician was that I could offer no treatment," he says, still remembering many of his first patients by name.

Truman has been treating leukemic children for nearly twenty-five years. Despite the emotional demands of his practice and his graying hair, Truman remains boy-

ish in appearance. And, in addition to retaining his
youth, he has held onto a characteristic physicians can
easily lose—their sensitivity to the human feelings that
attend life and death. Truman clearly comforts his patients while caring for them. Yet he retains a lively intellectual curiosity about the theories of medicine. When
asked if perhaps clinical physicians in the throes of administering treatment and arresting symptoms pay
enough attention to cause, he says thoughtfully, "That
is a good question because on one level, we think about
it all the time. In pneumonia, we immediately look for
a specific organism, a specific cause. But in another way,
we can be kind of rigid when we come to a disease that
has no known cause, like leukemia."

When Jimmy Anderson was diagnosed in 1972,
though John Truman had given Jimmy's parents some
hope in the prospect of treatment, the epidemiology of
leukemia was young, and there was little to go on by
way of cause. So noted Dr. Clark W. Heath, Jr., a veteran
investigator of clusters, who wrote a review chapter on
leukemia for the book *Cancer Epidemiology and Prevention.*

According to Heath, "effective epidemiologic studies" of leukemia began for the first time in the years
prior to World War II. Interestingly, it was again the
development of tools—in this case a language of disease
classification and the widened use of bone marrow as-
piration techniques—that made classic leukemia epidemiology possible. Before World War II, according to
Heath, scientists described the disease simply on the
basis of clinical "anecdotes"—what amount to personal
observations, often isolated, from which scientists be-

lieve little can be extrapolated. In fact, even today, to call a scientist's findings anecdotal is practically like calling it gossip in that it has not been verified and cannot yield further understanding.

The clinical anecdotes on leukemia, moreover, according to Heath, confused the real malignancy of the blood with a breakup of white blood cells brought on by infection.

Perhaps the first great breakthrough in developing theories about possible causes of leukemia was the medical aftermath of the research that brought us the atomic bomb. That leukemia could be associated with chronic exposure to ionizing radiation was first shown in 1944 in a study of radiologists who had excessive rates of leukemia and other blood diseases. Prior to this time, the dangers of radiation were not recognized or known and in fact many children in the 1930s and 1940s received intense radiation therapy to shrink enlarged thymus glands or to prevent the regrowth of recently removed tonsils. My own mother consented in 1949 to having the fetus she was carrying, me, irradiated to be sure I was in proper position for delivery. Since then we have learned such a procedure was foolhardy. No physician in America today would recommend a fetal x-ray examination as a routine matter.

In fact, in studies of children who had their throats irradiated, higher rates of thyroid and throat cancers have been observed. Early in the 1950s increased rates of leukemia began to be seen among survivors of the atom bomb blasts in Hiroshima and Nagasaki in 1945. Since then further studies have confirmed higher rates of most cancers among these survivors.

The viral theory had also been receiving much research attention through the 1960s as researchers began to explore the possibility that viruses caused human cancers. In fact, early cluster investigations, such as the one in Niles, Illinois, tested the viral theory, since the leukemias seemed to be grouped in proximity that would suggest contagion.

Leukemia viruses in animals, in particular, were being identified, and so science was engaged in attempting to discover whether genetic transmission of these viruses in humans could account for what Heath described as "familial tendencies" in the disease, or for the origins of the disease itself.

So when Anne Anderson asked the inevitable unanswerable question of her physician, "why Jimmy?" there were only two known environmental possibilities: radiation and viruses. Yet Jimmy had not been exposed to any extra radiation either before or after birth, and the virus theory was still inconclusive.

The potential involvement of chemicals was virtually unthought of at the time, at least in Jimmy's case. Benzene was the likeliest culprit, having been shown to be capable of causing leukemia us early as 1928 and of depressing bone marrow function as well as causing chromosomal damage. Humans were exposed in various industries, but also at home, since the strong solvent benzene was common in paint removers and paints, as well as in gasoline fumes.

In 1963 a United States Department of Health, Education and Welfare study reported a 54% increase in cancers of the blood among rubber industry workers who handled benzene. In 1964 shoe and rotogravure workers in Milan and Padua, Italy, who handled benzene were shown to be at higher risk of leukemia. And in 1972 a major study of Turkish shoe industry workers showed increased incidence of aplastic anemia—or depressed bone marrow function—and leukemia.

But no physician, including John Truman, mentioned benzene to the Andersons or asked about Jimmy's possible exposure to it. Nor did possible chemical exposures as a cause occur to Anne or Charles Anderson.

In one way the physicians could not be blamed. Benzene had so far been associated with myelocytic leukemia, not Jimmy's lymphocytic type. And the dangers of benzene were not known among laypersons, nor was the entire subject of chemical carcinogens much on the medical or public mind.

So there was really no answer for Anne Anderson, who continued to grasp for a reason. In her anguish she reviewed her own life habits. "Was it something defective in me that was carried on to him?" "Was it something I did wrong, something I gave him?"

But neither inside herself nor from those around her could Anne Anderson satisfy her question, and it paled in the face of the practical reality before her. She and her husband began the grueling business of caring for a gravely ill child. On the recommendation of Dr. Truman, they did not tell their other children about the seriousness of Jimmy's illness out of fear they were too young to understand and would themselves be afraid. Chuck was only five, but Christine, then nine, figured that Jimmy's illness had to be serious. She was told that because he had to be protected from germs, it would be best if she did not have her friends over to the house for awhile. Jimmy himself was still so young he could not yet even tell his parents when and where he hurt, or understand that the regimen of treatment on which he was about to embark was not the normal round of activity for a toddler.

Leukemia treatment consists of focusing powerful agents such as radiation and drugs on the renegade leukemia cells in the hope of eradicating them and of keeping others from developing. Jimmy was first treated with what was called the St. Jude's Protocol, named for the research hospital in Memphis, Tennessee, where it was developed. It called for a series of radiation treatments to the head area, a haven for leukemia cells, and several powerful drugs: methotrexate, a yellow pill; vincristine and prednisone, small white pills; and Cytoxan, a big speckled pill. Jimmy and his mother were gone so much of the time to Boston for these treatments that the neighbors later told Anne that before they knew of Jimmy's illness, they wondered if Anne and her son had moved out of the neighborhood.

News of Jimmy's illness spread among the Andersons' friends. First to know had been Carol Gray, Anne's lifelong friend, who herself had had three children by then. Gray provided the backbone of the network of people who began visiting, sometimes bringing over a cooked meal to spare Anne's preparing dinner, sometimes just providing a comforting presence. But too, these friends brought encouraging words, mostly that children with leukemia did survive. And, one friend offered, there was living proof right in Anne Anderson's neighborhood: two children with leukemia lived almost across the street from each other just a few blocks from the Andersons. They were Michael Zona, age seven, and another child whose parents to this day do not feel comfortable about publicizing their son's name.

Anne Anderson had not known about these cases, nor did she find their existence particularly comforting. A vague sense, partly fed by anger and confusion, began to build that somehow the cases were connected, reinforced by visits to the hospital during Jimmy's treatments and seeing other mothers in the waiting rooms, only to see them again within days on the streets of her own neighborhood. One morning in 1972 Anne Anderson remembers having noticed a woman putting out garbage on an East Woburn street, then seeing the woman at the hospital waiting for her own child to finish receiving his leukemia treatment.

They were women Anne Anderson did not know, and she was then unwilling and unable to approach them, being afraid they would think she was prying. And she recalls, "I knew that if they were like me, they would not really be able to talk about their child's leukemia very much. It is something you feel you should be keeping private."

But Anne Anderson began keeping mental notes too on the cases she observed, while plunging herself fully into the business of caring for Jimmy.

These were days of trips to Boston, twice a week sometimes, sometimes daily for injections or tests once Jimmy had been released from the hospital after his diagnosis. The trips were exhausting, but when Jimmy felt well enough to play, Anne wanted to let him. Jimmy adored snow and would ask to be allowed to go out. His mother, torn between her fear he would catch a cold and her wish to see him have some fun, packed extra sweaters into his snowsuit so that he looked, his sister says, "like a tiny blimp." But most often, bouts with the nausea and diarrhea that often accompany leukemia treatment kept Jimmy Anderson inside.

In the meantime, Anne Anderson became immersed not only in learning about what to expect from Jimmy's treatment for leukemia but in the disease itself. She and John Truman talked a lot about leukemia viruses and Anne read as much as she could on the subject. Slowly she began to think that maybe the foul water—which by 1972 had gotten no better in East Woburn—could perhaps be carrying such a virus or "germ" through East Woburn. She tested her theory on her husband, who found it doubtful, and on her friends, who did as well. Carol Gray, a friendly, warm woman who shared Anne's devotion to motherhood and family, was the only friend Anne had who did not outright discourage her theory that there might be a link between the leukemia cases. Gray thought Anne needed all the support she could get.

Anne Anderson herself knew that she was operating just on instinct, and without scientific training she felt somewhat at sea. When she questioned John Truman about the proximity of the cases, he simply said she was hearing about leukemia cases more than she had as a younger woman because people who knew Jimmy brought other cases to her attention as a means of comforting her and because children with leukemia were living longer and were therefore more apparent and obvious to everyone. Anne Anderson did not then know of the existence of the Centers for Disease Control, nor of the phenomenon of clustering.

She also did not know Patricia Kane, a nurse who with her husband, Kevin, and her children, Margaret, Kathleen, Timothy, and Kevin, Jr., lived in a blue-shingled, split-level house across Walker Pond from the Andersons, just barely in sight of the Anderson house.

Kevin Kane, Jr., was diagnosed with acute lympho-cytic leukemia in June 1973 at the age of two and a half. Patricia Kane had been one of the women Anne Ander-son had noticed at the hospital, but Anne did not know that the Kanes lived in East Woburn until one day when Carol Gray telephoned. Gray, not knowing that Anne had been noticing Pat Kane at the hospital, phoned with the news that another boy, Kevin, had been diagnosed with leukemia. Anne Anderson says, "I remember that call like it was yesterday. I thought 'my God' another one, and I was overwhelmingly sad and frustrated, mainly because it was happening again and I did not think it should have been happening." Shortly there-after, Anne Anderson saw Patricia Kane shopping at a market in Woburn.

The Kanes meanwhile too wrestled with the horrible reality of a potentially fatal disease striking their young-est child. He too had been put on the St. Jude's protocol; he too was in the care of John Truman. In 1973 Kevin received 176 treatment injections, more than one every other day, often administered to him at home by his mother.

Pat Kane, a devout Roman Catholic, is a sandy-haired woman who remembers trying to take Kevin's diagnosis in stride. She and her husband, a manager in a public utilities office in Boston, both grew up in Woburn and decided to stay on there. "At first," she says, "our reaction was grief and tears, and no matter what they tell you about a fifty-fifty chance of survival, you see your son with all those tubes in him and you just think he's going to be gone." All the Kanes could think of as they embarked on Kevin's treatment, besides hoping that their worst fears would be proven wrong, was that his disease was according to Patricia Kane, "just one of those things you can't understand because it can't be explained. One of those things you cannot do anything about."

Pat Kane eventually began noticing Anne Anderson too at the hospital, but the two women exchanged no more than the understanding knowing nods meant to comfort that pass between the relatives of patients in cancer treatment clinics. They would not meet for several more years.

The Kanes also experienced water problems. The water in their taps always smelled they say, often emitting that familiar rotten egg odor. It did not taste very good either. At some point after Kevin's diagnosis, the Kane's switched to bottled water, but not because they suspected any link between Kevin's leukemia and the water. The Kanes never made that connection, they admit, nor once they heard of Jimmy Anderson's case, did they make any connection between Kevin and Jimmy.

But Anne Anderson's analytical mind continued to knit events together, and her preoccupation, along with Jimmy's understandably central position, began to rock the keel of the family and household. When Jimmy was not feeling well, which was most of the time, Anne's attention was practically exclusively focused on him.

The two other Anderson children, Chris and Chuck,

were almost necessarily eclipsed, as Anne often had to leave them to amuse themselves while she threw herself into trying to comfort Jimmy who, weakened by the medication and the disease, could not play rough games or even be left alone very much. He sometimes vomited all day and night as a result of the drugs and had problems sleeping, so when he did at last slip into a nap, the other children had to be quiet, almost silent, in their own home. Family outings were often canceled at the last minute because Jimmy was too sick to go or because the money had been usurped by an emergency medical expense. Both Anne and Charles Anderson tried to make up for the extra attention paid to Jimmy to their other children, but balance was not easy to achieve.

Jimmy's need for constant care was also beginning to take a toll on the Anderson marriage. Anne Anderson's mental and physical energies were taken up almost entirely with caring for Jimmy while attempting to keep the household running and retain a few moments for herself—to keep up with news of the outside world or to just plain think. There were days she recalls when she almost dropped from exhaustion at supper time, so wracked was she by the unrelenting demands of Jimmy's illness, little sleep, and the competing list of things to do.

Charles Anderson too was tense. "There were just so many little extra pressures all the time on all of us. Not to mention extra expenses above the basic medical expenses." Money—for hospital visits, medicines, toys to keep Jimmy amused, outings for the other children, meals in restaurants to celebrate the end of a hospital ordeal—was constantly being spent. It was virtually impossible to keep to a family budget, and Charles Anderson, as earner of the family income, began to worry if he would be able to earn enough.

Also, he continued to have extensive business travel obligations, and when he came home, there was little time to talk of fun and less time to have any. Jimmy's condition became the measuring stick of married life. And the more Jimmy suffered, the angrier and more convinced Anne Anderson became that his illness might be related to the other leukemia cases, her concern a blend of speculation, fear, and frustration.

She became somewhat obsessed, she admits, insisting to her husband that something might have made Jimmy and the other children sick. Since Charles Anderson was away so much of the time, he heard of other cases only through Anne, and he simply did not perceive their bizarre proximity.

"As I insisted more," she describes, "we would argue. Charlie would say, 'you can't tell me that if these cases were unusual, somebody somewhere wouldn't be keeping an eye on them.'"

But nobody was. At the time there was no tumor registry in Massachusetts and no data being collected about how many cancer cases were being diagnosed, let alone where they were being diagnosed. There was no data to support Anne's instinct that the number of cases in such a small area was abnormal, even if she had known where to look for the data.

To attempt to help his wife come to more peaceable terms with Jimmy's condition, Charles Anderson, an active member of Trinity Church, asked the family pastor, Bruce C. Young, to counsel Anne. Young had been in-

strumental in helping Anne locate transportation in and
out of Boston to Massachusetts General. Anne did not
have a driving license because she had had no need to
drive a car really before Jimmy's illness. Charles Anderson, or friends, had driven her shopping or wherever
else she needed to go, but during the day when Jimmy
had to go to Boston for treatment, most people, including Charles Anderson, had to be at work. After Jimmy's
diagnosis, Anne simply could not find the time to take
the driving tests, and so she was essentially stranded.
Driving herself would have been impossible anyway, for
very often Jimmy, still only a toddler, needed to be held
in her arms during the trips, so uncomfortable did the
disease and its treatment make him.

Bruce Young asked around the church for people who
might drive her, and several parishioners pitched in. But
soon he began to find it easier to do the driving himself
rather than coordinate third parties. Charles Anderson
asked Young to take advantage of this time in the car,
back and forth to the hospital, to "talk Anne out of her
theories about the water," according to Young.

Young, a dark-haired man with an earnest full face,
had come to Woburn in 1966. He plays golf, drinks an
occasional martini before dinner, and tells good stories.
But he is a committed Christian who believes that spir-
ituality is founded on plain human decency and depends
on moral courage.

Bruce Young was born in Danvers, Massachusetts, in
1939 and moved to nearby Peabody early in his life,
which like Woburn depended on the tanning industry
for a good deal of its income. Young's father worked in
a leather factory; his uncle was a salesman for a com-

pany that sold leather finish, and some of his biggest customers were in Woburn. Young is acutely mindful that in his family "bread got put on the table by leather."

Because his parents felt he needed more discipline than he was receiving in the public schools, they enrolled him in a Roman Catholic preparatory school. But the rector of the Episcopal church was concerned that Bruce would lose sight of his own religious faith, and, as Bruce Young describes it, "he kind of took me under his wing." Attending Catholic school, Young became the protege of his minister and slowly got to see what the job was like.

Young says he didn't have a particularly fervent religious feeling but when he decided to attend Trinity College in Hartford, Connecticut, he began to think seriously about the ministry as a profession. He met his wife, Ruth, in the late 1950s, and the two were married in 1962.

By that time, Young had completed seminary training. He had gotten what he calls a "lucky draw" at a prestigious parish in New Canaan, Connecticut. He considers that a significant period in his life. He had been the first member of his family to attend college and had grown up unaware that affluence could create its own particular brand of social problem. He remembers talking with many male parishioners who had lost important jobs because of alcoholism. He heard for the first time about drug use among the well-to-do. He helped soothe the turmoil of families that seemed to be brought about by a lack of human sympathy, which money could not help.

When he graduated from the seminary program, Young took a job as an assistant curate in Attleboro,

Massachusetts. It was the time of the early civil rights marches in the South, and in 1964, Young's parish received an appeal from southern churches to send personnel to help with drives to register black voters. Young decided to volunteer, and he spent ten days traveling the back roads of McComb County, Mississippi, signing up black voters who were too intimidated to go into towns to register.

Just as Young had not grown up among the affluent, neither had he had an awareness of the severely depressed economic conditions of blacks in the South, or of the extent of rigid segregation. He was dumbfounded when he was warned that he and his friends should never be seen with blacks in the same car lest they be beaten up. "For the first time in my life," he said, "I learned that a representative of the law could be an enemy. It was a shock to me that the last person I wanted to meet in McComb if I was talking to a black person was a white policeman."

He and several other volunteers slept on floors in shacks in black communities, and he remembers that whenever they heard a car motor at night, they would roll away from the outside wall because they were so afraid that midnight riders were about to toss a bomb.

When Martin Luther King marched on Washington, Young was among the crowd, and he remembers being only about 150 feet away from King during the famous "I Have a Dream" speech. Recalls Young, "I did not realize then how much of history was being made at that moment. But I was incredibly moved by the sight of so many people, the feeling of the importance of the moment. It was a highlight of my life."

Bruce Young rejoined his wife in Attleboro and

brought the civil rights struggle home with him. He became active in the parish area, starting at the level of haircuts, for he gradually became aware that black people in Attleboro could find no one who would cut their hair. And while Young's parishioners were sympathetic with the civil rights movement, they thought of segregation as a southern phenomenon and were largely indifferent to the more subtle forms prevalent in the north.

He pointed out the haircut problem to the area cosmetology association in the hope the local barbers would become more sensitive to it. With modesty he says "I think we were pretty successful with that."

But Young did not think of himself as a rabble-rousing theologian. When he was offered the job as minister in Woburn, he accepted because he was interested in establishing an extensive Christian education program there. He liked the beautiful old church, with thick oak beams across the ceiling which creak on a windy day. He came to Woburn with his wife in the summer of 1966. She pursued her career in psychiatric work; their two sons were born; and the rest he says, "just sort of unfolded."

When he began driving Anne and Jimmy Anderson to and from the hospital, he simply put the driving in the good Samaritan category, along with his other ministerial jobs.

From the start, he doubted Anne's hypothesis that water might have caused the leukemia cases, he says as he looks across his cluttered desk over photographs of two of the children, including Jimmy. "It just seemed so unlikely," he recalls. But he felt that allowing Anne to express her feelings would be helpful to her. Young puts both hands on top of his head when considering life's ironies, and he says, "I decided the best therapy for Anne would be to get her involved in the information-gathering process, to really try to keep tabs on the cases. I thought sooner or later she would stop hearing of them."

By June 1975, Jimmy Anderson had received nearly three and a half years of therapy. In addition to the chronic diarrhea and vomiting, he had suffered hair loss, which he covered with a baseball cap, and had acquired a slight speech impediment and learning disability due to the radiation treatments, plus a deficiency in fine motor control. The therapeutic suppression of his white cell production left him vulnerable to infection, and in this period, he suffered pneumonia, frequent bronchitis, and constant fatigue, flus, and fevers.

Yet because his disease had come on so early Jimmy had not known another way of life. Therefore he never complained about the travails of the treatment or the limitations of his life because it was what he had come to think of as normal. He was not aware of the gravity of his illness, although he did know that it made him different in that it kept him from doing certain things that his older brother, Chuck, did as a matter of course. In fact, Jimmy now and then would watch from the windows as Chuck ran vigorously off to some game or athletic event. Then Jimmy would lose himself in drawing sailboats, across the sails of which he might write a message for his mother like "I Love You, Mom."

This constant reminder that Jimmy's life had been irrevocably changed fueled Anne Anderson on and put her in an almost classic position of a mother fighting for her young. In Anne's mind the villains were still somewhat vague, but they included the authorities who "dismissed my calls about the water because I was a housewife" and the medical establishment that could not answer her questions about whether the cases she was counting were too many. And also Anne Anderson, a shy, traditional woman with an untraditionally questioning mind, was beginning to perceive that her instincts were "just being put aside as the emotions of a mother." She began to feel the victim of an underlying sexism from which even her own husband was not immune.

She was being torn by loyalties—to conventional belief and faith in expert authority, to conventional feelings that a husband should take the lead, and to her own common sense and belief that her theory was worthy of at least some serious consideration. She did not have the epidemiology training of a John Snow, of course, but she had his hunch, and had she had his information about where the water to her home was coming from, she might have pulled the pump handle on well G and H, so to speak, and perhaps altered the course of Woburn's health history from that point on.

But she did not, and events continued.

Jimmy's first treatment protocol ended just before the summer of 1975. Jimmy survived the near fatal bout with chicken pox, and the family took their vacation and bought their cottage in Epping. Early that fall, however, they received the news that there were indeed leukemia cells in Jimmy's blood again. He was returned to chemotherapy.

Meanwhile, development continued full throttle at Industri-Plex, and water demand continued to expand in Woburn. In 1975 supplementary well G was pumping from May 17, 1975, until October 20, 1975; then again from November 18, 1975, through the winter to March 18, 1976. Well H came on in June 25, 1975, and stayed on until August 7, then pumped again from August 21 to September 10. And though it is impossible to be sure, it is likely that from the first days these wells came into operation, they were pumping water contaminated with toxic chemicals, while no one who drank it, washed with it, or complained about its taste and odor knew.

4

The Sea Underground

WHEN CHILDREN squat on their knees and start digging holes in the ground heading "to China," they will usually hit moisture, mud or water itself, if they dig long enough. Groundwater lies under the earth, a sea constituted of drops of water that fall as rain or snow or settle in the land as overflow from rivers, streams, and lakes.

According to the United States Water Resources Council, estimates of how much groundwater exists in the United States range from 33 to 100 quadrillion gallons. This accounts for 96% of the country's fresh water, or 16 times the volume of the Great Lakes. Lake Michigan alone contains 1,290 trillion gallons of water.

Often groundwater erupts on the surface as springs, streams, or lakes, and groundwater accounts for up to 30% of the surface in the western part of the United States.

About one half of all the people in the United States depend on groundwater for drinking. In rural areas the dependency rises to 95%. Use of groundwater for all purposes—drinking, washing, irrigation, and industrial processes—nearly tripled between 1950 and 1980, climbing from 34 to 88.5 billion gallons per day.

In Woburn, Massachusetts, until 1979 when the town joined the Metropolitan District Commission (MDC) water system, it had depended exclusively on wells dug into the Horn Pond and Aberjona aquifers. Aquifers are saturated underground layers, usually of sand or gravel, into which a well taps. They occasionally bubble up above the surface of the land in the form of a swamp or marsh, though most aquifers occur within 2,500 feet of the surface. The Aberjona aquifer in Woburn, which fed wells G and H, breaks the surface of the land to include the Aberjona River.

Some confined aquifers are simply sheets of underground water that could, in theory, be drunk with a straw if one could get a straw down into them. Under the Pine Barrens, for example, drifts of sand and blueberry bushes in New Jersey, according to writer John McPhee, there is an aquifer of clear, pristine water equivalent to "a lake seventy-five feet deep with a surface of a thousand square miles."

Groundwater moves through the layers toward gravity at less than a snail's pace, sometimes as slowly as a fraction of an inch a day but usually not faster than a few feet per day. The rate of movement depends on the pressure being exerted on the water by the layers and the permeability of each layer, in the way that how fast one can mop up a spill of water on a kitchen floor depends on whether one uses a sponge or a wad of typing paper. As gravity-seeking groundwater meets each layer, it flows through, under, or around as though negotiating an underground maze.

Once contaminated, groundwater cannot be easily cleaned, but almost more importantly, the contamination process cannot be monitored as it occurs because it takes place underground and, obviously, out of sight. Though groundwater was once an almost perfectly pristine resource, in the time span of one generation every state in the Union has developed some form of groundwater contamination serious enough to require the closing of some wells, sometimes wells on which millions of people depend. In February 1984 the General Accounting Office (GAO), the investigating arm of the United States Congress, issued a report on groundwater contamination that said, "although groundwater contamination is a significant and widespread problem, the extent of the contamination is unknown because no comprehensive national data base or monitoring program exists."

In 1983 the National Well Water Association estimated that about 1% of groundwater in the United States could be contaminated, which does not sound like much except that the contamination usually occurs in areas of dense population, and a small amount of contamination can affect a large number of people. For example, according to the Environmental Protection Agency (EPA), one single gallon of gasoline seepage into groundwater would be enough to jeopardize the drinking supply of a community as large as 50,000 people.

Leaking gasoline from underground storage containers at gas stations and supply depots (termed "LUSTs" by the EPA) account for a good deal of groundwater contamination. There may be as many as 75,000 to 100,000 faulty storage tanks leaking as much as 11 million gallons of gasoline annually according to EPA testimony in November 1983 provided to the United States

Senate Environment and Public Works Committee's Toxic Substances Subcommittee.

Septic tank leakage accounts for another 3.5 billion gallons of contamination each year, a dramatic example of which can be found in the rapidly developed counties of Nassau and Suffolk on Long Island near New York City, where wells serving 2 million people or more have been closed.

Agricultural pesticides also cause contamination, as poisonous chemicals that were used on the land are carried off by the rain and wind into the groundwater.

But perhaps the most worrying of the sources of groundwater contamination is toxic waste disposal practices. All of the 22,000 EPA-estimated known hazardous waste sites that consist of buried rusting barrels, or pits, ponds, and lagoons, have the potential to percolate like brewing coffee down into groundwater supplies. According to the February 1984 GAO report, "limited studies by the Environmental Protection Agency (EPA) and others conclude that groundwater contamination, particularly as a result of hazardous waste, is a serious national problem."

Toxic contamination travels underground in waves or "plumes," sometimes moving with water or behind it, or even getting ahead so it can lie in wait, so to speak. According to the National Science Foundation, a toxic plume—a collection of chemicals—"can widen and thicken as it travels and as more contamination leaches down with time."

For example, take the case of the Stringfellow acid pits near Riverside, California, a 22-acre tract that contains approximately 34 million gallons of toxic material dumped between 1956 and 1972 and that as of spring 1985 had yet to be cleaned up. A toxic plume seeped into local groundwater supplies, and in August 1984 a report by the Congressional Office of Technology Assessment warned that seepage was heading for the underground reservoir that supplies water to 500,000 people in Riverside and Los Angeles counties. California had spent $6 million studying ways to clean the acid pits and stop the groundwater contamination, and the EPA had budgeted $10 million more, but as of mid-1985, the problem had yet to be contained.

A similar leaching plume threatens the water supply of Atlantic City, New Jersey, and many other areas where millions of people live are subject to similar danger.

Even some of the largest waste landfills, areas where toxic wastes have been moved for supposedly safe disposal, supervised by the EPA have been found to be leaching their chemicals into the water underground. In November 1984, for example, the EPA was rocked by the news that a landfill operated by Cecos International, where many of the wastes excavated from Love Canal and other sites around the country were buried in what was thought to be a leakproof disposal facility, was itself leaking. Confusion laced the earliest reports, as at first the New York State EPA denied that the site was leaking, while an official of EPA headquarters in Washington, D.C., insisted that it was. Then, regional EPA officials suggested the problem originated not at the Cecos site but rather from an adjacent landfill operated by E. I. du Pont de Nemours Company. The du Pont wastes, it was argued, were leaking into the Cecos site, corroding the Cecos underground liners, causing the Cecos wastes to leak. On top of this, in an attempt to determine what was actually happening, investigators wore white safety suits and face masks as they tested for underground contamination, while their superiors were advising residents that there was "no danger" to the public from the landfills.

A certain amount of contamination is natural, particularly in arid areas where minerals can leach into the water from soil, or salts can concentrate in the water itself. It is usually the presence of salts and minerals that accounts for smelly and bad tasting water, especially for the "rotten egg" sulfur smell that can emanate from a tap the moment it is turned on, particularly in rural areas.

The relationship between contaminated drinking water and health problems is clear when the problem leads to dysentery or diarrhea akin to the dread Montezuma's revenge. However, the health effects of toxic chemicals in water in general are not well understood, nor are possible links to cancer in general or leukemia in specific. And though public awareness of the problem may be relatively recent, the problem is not. For example, as early as 1968 an article in the *Journal of the National Cancer Institute* reported that an unusually high number of skin cancer cases had been noted in Taiwan, Germany, and Argentina among users of particular wells contaminated with arsenic, a known cancer-causing substance also found at the Woburn Industri-Plex waste site in 1979.

In December of 1980 the President's Council on Environmental Quality issued a report entitled "Drinking

Water and Cancer: Review of Recent Findings and Assessment of Risks." The report reviewed and summarized relevant research on the subject and concluded, "recently completed case control studies have strengthened the evidence for an association between rectal, colon and bladder cancer and drinking water quality provided by the earlier epidemiological studies reviewed by the National Academy of Sciences committee. While the epidemiological studies completed to date are not sufficient to establish a causal relationship between chlorinated organic contaminants in drinking water and cancer, they do contain evidence which supports such a relationship for rectal cancer, and to a lesser degree, for bladder and colon cancer."

Most studies that attempt to determine the relationship between groundwater contamination and public health are hampered by the fact that, for the most part, groundwater contamination cannot be seen, smelled, or heard. As a National Science Foundation report on the subject noted in August 1983, "the tangible effects of groundwater contamination usually come to light long after the incident causing the contamination has occurred. The long time lag between occurrence and detection is a major problem, as irreversible damage may occur before the incident is discovered."

Such was the case in Woburn.

It seems likely that in the late 1960s and early 1970s when Anne Anderson and other East Woburn residents were complaining about their water, the objectionable smell and taste were being caused at least in part by high levels of salts and minerals, including iron and manganese in the water at the time. In June 1975, when the Massachusetts Department of Health wrote to the Woburn Water Board, suggesting that Woburn "treat" the wells, it was referring to the removal of these minerals and salts.

What no one at the Massachusetts Department of Public Health (MDPH) knew in 1975 was that the groundwater which fed wells G and H was also probably contaminated with toxic chemicals. In fact the entire matter of toxic wastes was yet unspoken. Love Canal had not yet happened, and the existence of toxic wastes in Woburn was known to no one.

But the MDPH and Woburn city officials had known since wells G and H began operating that the water they pumped would require chlorination. This was unusual in itself since it is normally surface water, not deep groundwater, that must be chlorinated against fecal contamination from sewers and septic tanks and other bacterial problems. However, when the first waters were sampled from G and H and found to contain bacterial contamination, it was assumed that because the wells were placed in a swampy area, decaying vegetation might have caused the problem. The MDPH permitted the wells to operate, provided the water was chlorinated.

At the time, chlorination was standard treatment meant to sanitize water. But in Woburn, chlorine reacted with the high mineral content, causing the manganese to precipitate. This is partly what was causing the brown spots on glasses and dishwashers throughout East Woburn. The request Woburn made in 1975 to change the chlorination system was largely to control the manganese problem by introducing still other chemicals that would hold the irksome mineral in solution.

But chlorination can have a further deleterious effect on water when chlorine meets organic substances in the soil, some of which may occur naturally. This interaction produces a group of chemicals known as trihalogenated methanes (THMs) such as bromoform, bromodichloromethane, and chloroform, a known carcinogen that was indeed present in the groundwater at Woburn, at least when the wells were finally tested in 1979. However, in a report on the analysis of Woburn well water prepared by a consulting engineering firm hired by the city of Woburn, Dufresne-Henry, dated January 1978, the possibility of THMs being present was not mentioned, although the chemical action of chlorine on naturally occurring organic matter was blamed in part for the tastes and odors.

The Dufresne-Henry report did, however, note something else.

With an eye toward eliminating the problematic chlorination altogether from wells G and H in 1977, the engineering firm had requested permission from state authorities to halt the chlorination of the wells on a trial basis. This was to determine whether the chlorine was reacting with "organic matter"—then assumed to be decaying vegetation—in the raw groundwater itself, or with groundwater stuck in the well distribution piping system. The engineers also wanted to determine what the yield would be in the G and H area should additional wells be sunk at a later time. Samples of the aquifer were taken at various points, and results were compared with those taken previously. One test well sunk between wells G and H showed many of the same salts and minerals as those two wells, but it also showed the presence of 2.79 milligrams per liter (mg/L) of carbon-chloroform extract (CCE), an umbrella term for organic chemical substances.

The CCE test had been in development in the late 1960s, and in the early 1970s it was the only method available for determining what organic substances were in water apart from bacteria. A basic CCE test could not say which specific substances made up the overall extract. However, the CCE test was at least a broad indicator that there could be problematic organic contamination, including chemical, in water.

Because the CCE test was time consuming and because for a while there was a possibility that the procedure was going to be adopted by the federal government as a method to use in determining drinking water standards, an enterprising chemical engineer at the Massachusetts Department of Environmental Quality Engineering (DEQE) laboratory, Al Silvia, set about researching a method that would be faster. He developed a fluorescence "surrogate" technique that could be done in a matter of hours, instead of the seven to nine days the test had taken up to that point.

The implications of Silvia's work were startling. For it meant that the state of Massachusetts would have at hand a rapid method for general water assays. Silvia's immediate superior understood the importance of the work Silvia had done, but the two engineers knew that they would have to verify that the experimental rapid CCE method was comparable to the old. So they decided to compare earlier CCE results to those to be collected with the new method, and by way of perfecting his new technique, Silvia received permission to use it in an ambitious plan to sample the water in every well in Massachusetts. He did it.

In April 1975 he sampled the water in Woburn. His results were quite dramatic. The wells in the Horn Pond area of southwest Woburn had CCE readings ranging from 0.42 to 0.63 mg/L, which was in keeping with other cities. However, wells G and H had CCE readings of 1.3 and 2.0, respectively. In retrospect Silvia says that readings like these would certainly have seemed "kind of high to me," but he adds, "at the time, I was doing research only on the method, and nobody knew much yet about how serious water contamination problems could be."

The CCE test was not specific enough to say exactly what contaminants could be in the water, and it picked up only nonvolatile organic chemical substances, not the volatile substances found later with more sophisticated methods. But Silvia's early Massachusetts surveys did point out some interesting trends, namely that CCE levels in public water tended to get higher as one moved from west to east in the state, which is the direction of industrialization and which also is the trend of contamination seen in the 1980s with more advanced testing procedures.

However, the CCE surveys, though they were of interest for what they suggested about Massachusetts water quality, tended to be viewed as important mostly for their verification of the reliability and viability of the rapid CCE technique. Silvia says he felt at the time that the tests showed he was "onto something," with respect to Massachusetts water quality, but he adds, "Nobody knew much what to do with the results and what they could mean, I guess."

Silvia also even remembers being called to a meeting about places where he found high CCE levels, such as Woburn, but that the questions had been to find out whether the results could have been false positives due to flaws in the test method. Silvia says, "I assured everybody they were not," but as Richard Chalpin, also of the DEQE, would later say about the general focus of scientific and administrative thinking at the time, "they were playing with a different sheet of music then." Toxic contamination of groundwater was not yet on the score.

The letter sent in June 1975 from the state of Massachusetts to the Woburn Board of Health about wells G and H made no reference at all to Silvia's April 1975 CCE results. However, the letter the state sent to the city in 1977, responding to the engineering firm's request to temporarily halt the chlorination of the water, did mention the CCE test that had been taken that year but did not specify what the level was or what it meant.

It was this 1977 result, of 2.79 mg/L CCE in the test well near wells G and H, to which the engineering consulting firm referred in its 1978 report. To explain the significance of the CCE results of the city, the Dufresne-Henry report said of the substances that would have made up the extract, "These organic contaminants—natural substances, insecticides, herbicides and other agricultural chemicals—are present in the groundwater of the Aberjona River Valley. Both natural and man-made contaminants can have undesirable effects on health and can cause tastes and odors. CCE in well water should not exceed 0.1 mg/L."

According to P. E. Pittendreigh, who wrote the engineering report, at the time he was unaware that CCE tests had been done in 1975, and consequently he did not know that the results in 1977 to which he was referring in his report were even higher than those found in the earlier tests.

The engineering report did note that the test well sunk in 1977 was fed by the same aquifer as wells G and H but did not explicitly say that therefore CCE was probably present also in those two wells. Nor did the report elaborate on the effects on human health that chemicals indicated by the CCE finding might have, nor highlight that the level in the aquifer test was well above the acceptable limit. But that CCE was present in the groundwater was the first indication that "man-made" organic chemicals might be part of the problem of wells G and H, and indeed it was the first indication—a year and a half before May 1979—that there could be chemical contamination of the Aberjona aquifer itself.

Dufresne-Henry pointed out that to remove the CCE "will require filtration through carbon," and it recommended that Woburn install an activated carbon "polishing" filter system on wells G and H. It also recommended a more orthodox sand filtering system, which would remove most of the problematic iron and manganese. The engineering firm stated that such a system would, in the long run, be less costly than full dependence on MDC water.

And it pointed out that while the city was not bound

by law to treat wells G and H with carbon, it would have to do so if it were to dig a new well in the same aquifer. In short, the aquifer had two problems: (1) iron and manganese and (2) CCE, which could have been indicating the presence of chemical contamination.

But in transit these two problems blurred into one.

The covering "letter of transmittal" accompanying the report from the engineering firm to the city of Woburn makes no reference to the CCE finding in the report and does not call attention to it. There is also no mention of the CCE finding in a summary of the report dated March 1978 by the Woburn Department of Public Works. This summary listed events chronologically in the background of the problems of wells G and H, but it included no reference of any kind to the presence of chemical contamination hinted at by the CCE finding.

The meat of the engineering report was, according to the summary, that "it will be necessary to treat the water from this field, and the [engineer's] estimate for this plant is $1,500,000."

That the engineer's report had actually advocated two types of treatment, one for CCE and one for minerals and salts, was also lost in transit.

It is likely that only the letter of transmittal and the summary, rather than the full engineering report, were ever read by those for whom the report had been intended. Robert W. Simonds, Public Works superintendent of Woburn, was assistant superintendent at the time and very involved in the discussion of what to do about wells G and H. In 1985, on having his attention called to the paragraphs referring to CCE, he said, "I do not recall any discussion within public works at the time of that specific item," meaning CCE and what it suggested. And he added, "I think when the mayor was making his decision [not to treat the wells], he was just looking at cost—he wasn't thinking about what kind of treatment it was going to be."

The mayor indeed decided not to install the treatment system on the basis of its cost. Robert Simonds said "it is just as well because it would not have gotten the toxic chemicals out anyway." That, according to the Dufresne-Henry report, is incorrect. A carbon filtration system aimed at nonvolatile organics such as those in the CCE would have grabbed volatile organics too, even though no one knew volatile organics to be present at the time. Mayor Higgins, for his part, declined to be interviewed for this book.

Since Woburn city officials maintain that the city never knew before May 1979 that there were chemical contaminants in the wells, it means that the significance of the CCE finding—that the Aberjona aquifer was potentially contaminated with man-made substances—was either not understood or ignored. At the least, a real response to the CCE finding would have been to make further inquiry about what it actually meant. True, the CCE finding did not predict the types of chemicals that were found in 1979, but on its own it was warning that synthetic substances were in the aquifer, and the Dufresne-Henry report made crystal clear what those substances could be. Moreover, Silvia was then at work on a technique that could have made the CCE method sensitive to a class of volatile organics similar to those found in 1979. In short, research was getting closer, and those who would have looked further probably would have found.

All this meant that the instincts of Anne Anderson and others who were complaining about bad water in their homes were actually not far from anticipating the chemical contamination that was eventually discovered. Clearly, chlorination of wells G and H from the outset had a lot to do with the complaints about the water, but it may also have been creating THMs in the system, like chloroform, and exacerbating the water's other smells and odors when it reacted with organic substances of the CCE type. Though the foulness of the water that bothered East Woburn residents in the late 1960s and early 1970s might have been nothing more than salts and minerals, no one can say for sure.

Moreover, while the water continued to be bad, information and clues were available that were not seized upon by those responsible for protecting water quality. The April 1975 findings, when wells G and H were tested and found to have high CCE levels, never got further than the research log of the enterprising chemical engineer who had collected them. Two years later the CCE readings in the aquifer were higher, but that there had been an increase was not perceived because nobody had all the pieces of the story, and so no one thought to look for a comparison.

Then in January 1978 the finding of CCE and the reference to chemical contamination in the aquifer that it could represent elicited no action. Thus the chemical history of wells G and H slipped into oblivion.

Had the city perceived the significance of the CCE findings as described to it by the engineering report it had contracted, it would have known that the Aberjona aquifer was potentially seriously contaminated—at the least with pesticides and insecticides—as of early 1978. But instead the town continued operating wells G and H untreated, and in fact well G operated continously through 1978, rather than in the summer months alone.

5

Unexpected Effects

ACCORDING TO reporter Michael Brown in his book *Laying Waste*, in 1977 a young woman took the microphone at a public meeting in Niagara County, New York, to protest the establishment of a landfill intended to receive toxic wastes generated by chemical producers in the area. She recounted her own personal knowledge of the effects of toxic waste to fortify opposition to having more hazardous substances piling up in the vicinity. Through her tears she spoke the words "Love Canal," describing how wastes from that dump site were already destroying her neighborhood, leaking into basements of homes and frightening residents, even making them and their children sick.

Brown says he at first discounted the woman's testimony, feeling that her "reaction had been based more on emotion than on facts." But Brown grew increasingly involved in the Love Canal saga, and by August 1978 when New York State ordered the emergency evacuation of 240 families, the small and modest neighborhood had become front page news around the country, a national symbol of the growing awareness of the problem of what to do with toxic wastes.

It took the dramatic disclosures about Love Canal to

write this new national music, as Richard Chalpin would put it, setting forth the environmental dilemma posed by the accumulation of toxic wastes. And all the shock would suggest that no one had ever heard of such environmental problems prior to the 1978 public revelations about Love Canal. But as early as 1962, in *Silent Spring*, Rachel Carson had written of the dangerous effects of toxic pesticides once sprayed lingering on in the soil, air, and water, upsetting the earth's natural balances with unexpected side effects. In the 1960s there was a flowering of the environmental movement; a switch flipped on in the consciousness of the world, flashing the message that it was time to begin stewarding and caring for natural resources after some 2,500 years of consuming and using them. In many respects, problems such as Love Canal and Woburn represent are simply chits being called in on bad practices of the past.

According to the federal Environmental Protection Agency, approximately 80 billion pounds of toxic waste is generated each year in the United States compared with about 1 billion pounds annually in the years following World War II. And, as it turns out, we produced this waste, indeed drastically increased our production of it, without any clear idea of where and how we would dispose of it or of the fact that we might be poisoning our water and land in the process. However, the possibility of poisoning was known at least to some well prior to the Love Canal incident.

One of the earliest cases of extensive pollution from toxic waste disposal practices came dimly to light in 1964 when thousands of fish in the muddy Mississippi River from Memphis to New Orleans floated to the river surface, dead. According to the book *Hazardous Waste in America*, by Dr. Samuel S. Epstein, Lester O. Brown, and Carl Pope, the fish kill was traced to the presence of contaminating organochlorine pesticides, such as endrin, which had their source in a toxic waste dump called Hollywood operated on the river shores near Memphis by the Velsicol Chemical Corporation.

Apparently, during heavy rains and high water periods on the river, water sloshed into the dump, dissolving solid waste residues from the production of pesticides, and then sloshed back into the river to kill the fish. Without acknowledging that this process had occurred, however, and without being subject to any irrefutable proof of a link between the waste dump and the fish kill, Velsicol nevertheless ceased using the Hollywood dump and moved its operation in August of 1964 to a 242-acre farm in remote Hardeman County, Tennessee. The site was approximately 50 miles east of Memphis and about 10 miles north of the rural town of Bolivar, off what is locally called the Toone-Teague road. Neither the family selling the land, the Fradys, nor their neighbors knew that the previously productive farmland would be used as a chemical dump.

The chemical wastes were shipped by truck in metal barrels, which were then rolled off into several unlined trenches and covered with dirt according to the then common "shallow burial" practice. The farm land chosen for the site was very permeable and sat on a lot of groundwater, groundwater that fed both the surface aquifer which supplied local wells and the deeper aquifer which provided drinking water to the 600,000 or so residents of Memphis. No precautions were taken to

keep the highly caustic materials from eating through
the barrels, which they did, and leaching into the soil
and water, which they also did. And there were no regulations that required such precautions be taken.

However, in March 1965 an alert individual, county
engineer Everett Hardof, according to *Hazardous Waste
in America,* pointed out the potential hazard from the
dump to the Tennessee Stream Pollution Control Board.
As a result, from 1966 to 1967, at the request of the state
of Tennessee, the United States Geological Survey
(USGS), an arm of the federal Department of the Interior, tested and found groundwater contamination had
indeed occurred around the Toone-Teague road dump
and had already reached water 90 feet below the surface.
Though the USGS stated that the contamination was
likely to persist because of the nature of the soil in the
vicinity, which allowed contamination to wander freely
through it, the USGS did not believe the chemicals could
seep 200 feet further to the deeper aquifer on which
Memphis was dependent. The USGS also concluded that
the contamination was traveling east, that is, away from
the local residential wells, which drew on the more shallow aquifer.

Velsicol expanded its practices, but during 1970 and
1971, another alert individual, a hydrologist with the
USGS, E. J. Kennedy, reopened the question of whether
the dump site was safe. In reviewing the predictions of
the 1967 water survey, Kennedy found their reliability
doubtful. More residential development had taken place
near the site, with concomitant need for more wells,
which drew more water. And the dumping had been so
extensive that it had seriously altered the quality of the

land and the natural flow of the groundwater. In fact, Kennedy found that the 1967 survey had greatly under-estimated the potential for contamination and misread the direction of the contaminant flow. The contamination was not traveling east at all, and local residential wells were indeed in jeopardy.

When Velsicol would not voluntarily cease dumping toxics at the Hardeman County site after being pre-sented with the revised USGS findings, it was ordered to do so by the state of Tennessee. Velsicol, however, continued its use of Hardeman County until 1975, when it finally closed the site after having dumped some 16.5 million gallons of water in 250,000 55-gallon drums.

There was not much national attention paid to the Hardeman County incident in the 1970s. Nor was much notice taken of events in the Minneapolis area, specifi-cally in St. Louis Park, which was not yet a full-fledged suburb. In 1961 the Reilly Tar and Republic Creosote Company opened a manufacturing facility on 80 acres, at which it produced creosote, a toxic wood preserva-tive, along with other wood preservatives and noxious chemicals, in a distillation process that gave off vapors of tars, oils, and gas.

In 1932 residential growth in St. Louis Park was under way, and the town hoped to meet the increasing water demand from the growing population by drilling a new 540-foot-deep well. But when the first water began spurting up through the well, it had to be condemned by the state health department because of creosote con-tamination. Preexisting wells in the area were then also tested, found to also be contaminated with creosote, and closed.

Preliminary investigations revealed that some of Reilly's waste-holding tanks had been leaking the manufacturing residue substances, but Reilly did not change its disposal systems. In fact, Reilly even deliberately emptied the overflowing dump tanks onto the ground in order to make room to fill them up again with new wastes. By 1957 the wells Reilly drew on to provide water to make its products were also found to be contaminated with manufacturing by-products, self-poisoned, as it were, and Reilly began buying water from the city because its own water was no longer pure enough to use.

St. Louis Park continued to develop, and Reilly continued its operations despite its tank and water problems. But in 1962 the mayor of Minneapolis, citing continuing problems of contaminated water in the vicinity, including run-off from rain, asked Reilly in 1962 to close the facility within ten years. The plant did close in September 1971, but not without there having been extensive additional contamination of the land and water with creosote, phenols, and other poisonous petroleum by-products, unbeknownst to the city of Minneapolis. However, the city did agree to take over title of the land from Reilly in the hope of developing it under a federal Department of Housing and Urban Development grant. Reilly asked to be "held harmless" for any liability for damages that might be incurred once the land changed title.

There was protracted legal battling between the city and the state as to whether Reilly could be relieved from costs incurred in cleaning up the site or for pollution of air or surface water. When this matter was finally settled in 1973, with the city agreeing not to hold Reilly liable, the city discovered that the land it had gone to much trouble to acquire was so saturated with creosote it could not be used at all, and moreover the municipal wells were found to be contaminated to depths of 900 feet. In short, the city of Minneapolis had acquired a giant mess.

The most notorious waste "discovery," Love Canal, burst full force into the news in 1978, but even it was not entirely unanticipated. Between 1947 and 1952, the Hooker Chemical Company had been dumping deadly chemicals such as lindane, a highly toxic pesticide; chlorobenzenes, derivatives of benzene; and trichloro-phenol (TCP) used in the manufacturing of pesticides, itself contaminated with tetrachlorodibenzo-para-diox-in (TCDD), otherwise known simply as dioxin, one of the most toxic substances in the world and one of the most potent known carcinogens. According to Samuel Epstein and others, several ounces of dioxin would be enough to kill the entire population of New York City, and there were several hundred pounds of it dumped by Hooker in Love Canal, making up part of a grand total of 21,800 tons of chemicals dumped over a five-year period.

In 1953 the Niagara Falls Board of Education, seeking land on which to build a new school it believed the community needed, eyed the Love Canal area. By then the canal itself had been filled in, and the board of education hoped to build a school on the new land. The board also expected that private and public developers would begin work on adjacent homes and other neighborhood facilities. Hooker, of course, knew what substances lay in and around the dump and offered to give the land to the school board for the token sum of $1 in exchange for a provision in the deed which stipulated Hooker would have no liability if the site should later prove unsuitable for building. In the transaction, Hooker disclaimed responsibility for any untoward effects that might be later tied to the site, but Hooker did not specifically warn the board about the dangers inherent in constructing anything, let alone a school, on such toxically saturated land.

The board began construction on the school and a playground, and a neighborhood indeed began to develop. In fact, when during the building of the school workers digging down hit a foul-smelling pit, the board simply ordered that the foundation for the school be moved 85 feet to the north, unaware of the extent and the nature of the materials that were in the canal and seeping underground, and were disinclined to investigate further. Also unaware were the people who lived in the vicinity.

In *Hazardous Waste in America* the authors quote a long-time area resident who remembers that she and other children had always called the Love Canal "quicksand lagoon." Of this resident's innocent relationship with the waste dump, the authors write, "She and her playmates poked sticks into the surfacing drums of chemicals and skipped rocks over the black sludge that accumulated there. The rocks popped and smoked as they bounced."

As early as 1957, when Hooker learned that the school board expected to sell some of the land directly to private residential developers, one of the company's attorneys sent an unelaborated message suggesting to the board that the site might not be suitable for residential construction. It was not until the chemicals literally began oozing through basement walls that the board learned why Hooker had sent that message and the menace of Love Canal became public knowledge, approximately thirty years after the dumping began.

There were other toxic problems brewing around the country prior to 1975, when Woburn was testing its wells for minerals, salts, and bacteria. In May 1971 in Moscow Mills, Missouri, at a horse-breeding ranch called Shenandoah Stables, road oil was sprayed in the training arena to hold down dust. Judy Piatt, co-owner of the ranch, had gone into the barn to feed and water the horses, and she noticed a strong smell coming up from the arena floor. She put the smell out of her mind and continued the chores. The next day there were sparrows falling dead from the barn rafters to the arena floor, and in the next few weeks, ranch cats and dogs died after losing their hair, growing thin, and constantly howling or crying.

Of eighty-five horses exposed to the arena, forty-three died within a year. Of forty-one newborn horses, only one survived. And on August 23 of 1971, Judy Piatt's own daughter was hospitalized with severe internal bleeding after having been complaining of headaches and nausea.

There are various sources of waste oil, that is, used oil, in the United States, and a major one is crank case oil drained from auto engines everywhere and then discarded. It was eventually discovered that the waste oil used to spray the arena had not been oil alone. Rather, it had been mixed with solid waste residue of TCP. The dealer, it seemed, also worked as a waste hauler and had been contracted to remove TCP and other wastes from a petrochemical plant in Verona, Texas. The dealer picked up his load, drove it to St. Louis, and dumped it in his tanks, which already contained waste oil. He then sprayed the lethal mix at Shenandoah Stables and elsewhere.

When samples from the Shenandoah Stables arena were sent to the federal Centers for Disease Control in Atlanta in August 1971, the precise chemical combination could not be specifically identified. Partly this was because the mass spectrometer gas chromatograph was not in use there yet, and so it was not until three years later, in 1974, that it became known that the main contaminant in the oil had been the deadly TCDD—dioxin. The same year the federal Environmental Protection Agency (EPA) issued a report on the problem of pollution from waste oil which said, in part, that the EPA had no idea where or how 31% of all the waste oil in the country was discarded.

The contaminated arena oil story eventually became a nightmare for the entire state of Missouri, culminating over a decade later in the federal government's having to evacuate and buy out entire contaminated towns, such as Times Beach, Missouri.

Also in 1971, as the horses, sparrows, barnyard animals, and children became sick at Shenandoah Stables in Missouri, the state of New Jersey had to close the Lipari landfill in Mantua Township. This was a 16-acre site located at a former gravel pit bordered by pretty peach and apple orchards, as well as two streams, one of which feeds the Delaware River. Within 100 yards of the landfill was a suburban residential development.

In 1958, although the land was purchased as part of a sand and gravel business, the owner also accepted toxic wastes for disposal in the deep earthen pits and continued doing so until 1971. Years after the site was closed the federal EPA discovered that approximately 3 million gallons of poisonous liquids were disposed on 6 acres at Lipari, though the materials seeped into another 10 acres, contaminating 49 million gallons of groundwater and 290,000 cubic yards of soil, plus 50,000 cubic yards of soil along the bordering streams. Again, these details on the extent of the contamination came to light years after the site was shut down. In 1971 it was only complaints from local residents about the odor, dying vegetation, and their own general sicknesses like headaches and nausea that brought official attention to the nature of business at the Lipari landfill.

While these and other troubling incidents were taking place around the country, the federal Congress was flushed with success in having passed major environmental legislation intended to protect the nation's air and water, albeit surface water, from pollution. However, these bills, the Clean Air Act passed in 1970 and the Clean Water Act passed in 1972, dealt only with emissions from factories and plants, those fumes and discharges that are coughed or spurted freely into the environment during manufacturing or production processes. The acts did not address themselves to pollutants that never survived long enough to be emitted, the bona fide waste that had to be taken out of the manufacturing stream earlier on.

In 1970 the Congress had passed the Solid Waste Act,

which intended to address the matter of wastes, such as garbage and sewage. However, it did not provide any regulation of hazardous toxic waste, but instead mandated a congressional level study of the toxic disposal problem. The study, however, was not submitted to Congress until four years later, and 1974 came and went without any legislative movement at the federal level on the hazardous waste problem.

At the time, few states had any legislative controls in place either, although Texas, the largest producer of hazardous waste in the country, did have a pertinent law on the books as early as 1969. Ironically it was partly to comply with this law controlling waste disposal that the Verona, Texas, waste producer had sold his wares to the hauler headed for Shenandoah Stables.

So in terms of both public awareness and legislative initiative, in 1975 when wells G and H were being tested in Woburn, the problem of toxic waste was on the national back burner, so to speak.

Scientists, for their part, also had priorities elsewhere. One of the first studies of the relationship between cancer rates and drinking water was published in *Science*, the scholarly journal, early in 1976. It found an excess mortality from gastrointestinal cancer among residents who drew drinking water from the Mississippi River, but possible links to chemical residues in the water were not explored.

Like the toxic substances migrating under the earth, awareness of their extent and potential impact on human health was bubbling but had not yet burst onto the national scene. It would take the public spectacle of families being evacuated from Niagara Falls and Love

Canal, New York, to tie together events such as the Mississippi fish kill of the mid-1960s and dumps in Tennessee and Missouri and New Jersey and indeed all across the nation. In 1975, when it was minerals and salts in wells G and H that had caught official notice, Anne Anderson had not heard of Toone-Teague road, or St. Louis Park, or the chemicals TCP, or TCDD, or TCE, and neither had any of the other parents whose children were, one by one, being diagnosed with leukemia.

The Quirk of Discovery

DONNA ROBBINS WAS BORN in northeast Woburn on October 9, 1949, one of twin girls. She remembers a typical childhood and particularly liking to play outdoors, climbing trees and generally enjoying what were then the open spaces of Woburn.

Hall's Field was a favorite spot with Donna Robbins and her friends, full of high marsh grass in which to hide and seek and veined with a small brook from which the children would often drink when they were not catching snakes in its waters. The children would also pick up what they called "mudpacks" and throw them at each other to see if they could break the thick, cracked chunks of earth into fragments. Donna and the others, of course, did not know that Hall's Field had been used as a chemical dump, that the packed "mud" was really congealed chemical residue, or that Hall's Brook was doubtlessly also carrying the wastes of many years of dumping.

Hall's Field was not far from the fields that have now become Industri-Plex, and the children also took for granted lands that have long since been condemned, riding their bikes all through the areas now part of the Industri-Plex waste site.

Donna Robbins graduated from high school in 1967,

met her former husband, and was married two years later. She moved into an apartment down the street from her mother's home in northeast Woburn. This period in her life, she remembers, was marked by memories of keeping windows closed. In 1972 she had a job as a bookkeeper with a company near what is now Industri-Plex, and while construction was underway, the office windows had to be shut to fight off the offensive odors that were beginning to emanate as contaminated lands and piles of hides that had been left undisturbed were suddenly hitting fresh air.

She was not relieved from odors at home either, for across the street, Hall's Field was also being dug up to create a new housing development. And always, the water, both at Donna Robbins' mother's and her own apartment, was foul. These houses both were within the reach of wells G and H. And when Donna and her husband, Carl, used to visit his family in Alabama, they would note immediately how lovely tasting the water was compared to that of home.

Carl W. Robbins, Jr., Robbie, was born March 15, 1972. He was a happy, normal baby. He was bottle fed, and by that time tapwater conditions had greatly deteriorated. Donna Robbins remembers even boiling water for cooking vegetables before using it, so foul and scummy was the water.

In 1974 Robbie developed a serious rash that lingered for two months. His pediatrician prescribed a salve, and when that did not work, he referred Donna Robbins to a dermatologist. The specialist was at a loss to determine the cause of the rash, but Donna Robbins remembers his having said, "All I can think is that there is something in his environment." Indeed, Hall's Field was still being excavated, and when at last the digging stopped, Robbie's rash disappeared.

Around this time too, however, the developer of Industri-Plex, D'Annolfo, began selling mounds of "earth" that had been moved off the site literally dirt cheap. The Robbins' landlord bought some and used it to landscape the Robbins' backyard. The toddler Robbie would play there, sometimes carrying along a bottle of water to drink.

When Robbie was two years old, the family moved into another apartment, a bit further from Industri-Plex, but still plagued by bad water in the taps. Kevin Robbins was born six months after the move, in January 1975.

The following summer in July, Robbie, then four and a half, toddled into the kitchen and told his mother he had pain in his groin. From one day to the next, Robbie could not comfortably walk, and he had begun to run a high fever.

His pediatrician examined him, suspected a septic hip inflammation, and told Donna Robbins that surgery was necessary to aspirate the joint. "All of a sudden," she says, "about an hour later, there was my son lying on a stretcher in a hospital. It's just awful to suddenly see your child like that, and he is going one way and you can't follow him. You just have to think his life is in their hands now."

During the surgery, Robbie's sciatic nerve was severed. This left him with permanent damage, necessitating that for the rest of his life, he wear a cast from his ankle to his hip and a special shoe to support his foot. Now faced with this as a prospective lifetime condition,

Robbie was released from the hospital. But the joint pain did not disappear. Within several days of his release, his other hip began to ache, then his arms and hands. His jaw was so sore he could not chew. He could not even roll over in bed alone, and his mother would do it for him so that he could fall asleep. Throughout the summer Robbie underwent tests, and still the pain did not subside.

On October 12, 1976, Donna Robbins was holding Robbie in her arms, comforting him in a favorite rocking chair. The phone rang, and it was her physician reporting the results of some additional blood tests that had been done on Robbie. "I guess they had been suspecting leukemia all along, but just never told me until they were sure. But that call—sure enough they were there, leukemia cells."

Until that point, Donna Robbins had distantly known the Andersons through church. Donna Robbins recalls, "I used to see Anne there with Jimmy, with his bald head, and I knew what he had. But I could never even talk to Anne and say 'well how is he doing' because you just don't know how to approach somebody about something serious like that. But then Robbie was diagnosed, and it was like night and day. I thought, 'Here is someone who knows what I am going through.'"

The two women began to become friends. Anne Anderson did not broach the subject of the water or her theories that the leukemia cases could be connected at first. She says, "I just did not know myself if I was crazy, and I didn't feel right involving another woman who was just beginning to go through that most difficult period when the diagnosis is new."

Donna Robbins says, "Anne gave me a lot of support.

There was that closeness, because these are things you can only talk about with someone in exactly the same circumstances. Sometimes it is only other mothers who know what it feels like when you find out your child might be going to die."

Prior to Robbie's diagnosis, the Robbins' marriage had been growing more strained, but the couple made an attempt to reconcile for the sake of Robbie and his brother. However, the attempt did not work, and Donna Robbins decided to end the marriage there and then. Divorce proceedings began shortly after Robbie's diagnosis. Donna Robbins took care of her two sons by day, and then with babysitting help from her mother and sisters, enrolled in nursing school at night. "I knew if I was going to be alone," she said, "I would need some kind of skill. And also I needed something to keep me from thinking about the leukemia because when I did, I fell apart."

Like Jimmy Anderson, Robbie had leukemia of the acute lymphocytic type, and he began a chemotherapy protocol supervised by his physicians at the Tufts University Medical Center. He began to experience the ups and downs of the treatment cycle. So did his mother.

"I wanted to have a lot of hope, but for some reason, I was scared to have too much because when things were going well with Robbie, and I got hopeful, then he would start feeling bad again. I had to stay away from that magical thinking."

With Robbie's diagnosis, Bruce Young's resistance to the idea that something was unusual in Woburn began to shake somewhat.

He had been listening to the steady drumbeat of

Anne's theories as the two rode in and out of Boston with Jimmy. They were making the trip so often that they could read the traffic patterns like experts and predict down to the minute how long the trip would take each day.

After Young quietly let Anne talk, he would attempt to battle her with his own brand of firmness: "Every now and then after she had made a point I would say, 'but Anne you need some kind of proof.'" That would deflect Anne Anderson's adamance somewhat and focus her on what she could do to shore up her instinct.

For her part, Anne Anderson valued even Young's superficial involvement at this point. For whenever she talked about the leukemia cases—she had heard of roughly ten cases by mid-1976—she would be seized again with the urge to do something, but she also faced a psychological and practical barrier that, alone and untrained in epidemiology, she did not feel equipped to scale.

The Robbins diagnosis was the second in the Trinity Church parish. Since Bruce Young had not expected there to be more cases, when he received the news of Robbie's leukemia he felt torn between a gut sense that the number of cases was strange and an awareness that they could all nevertheless be coincidental.

He says, "With Robbie the situation did begin to feel odd to me, but I didn't know if it was that same sensation as when I started all of a sudden noticing lots of Volvos on the road after I had bought one."

To reconvince himself there was nothing wrong, he telephoned the state public health department, he says, and asked if there were any investigations under way in

Woburn. He was told, he recalls, that no investigations were under way because there was nothing odd taking place to warrant investigating. He welcomed the reassurances, he remembers, taking them on faith.

In the meantime, in between caring for Jimmy, Anne Anderson did indeed attempt to gather "proof" in the only way she knew. Night after night, she went over her information on the leukemia cases. She had some names written on index cards, some on plain slips of paper. If she grouped the cases by school, there were four in the same small elementary school. If she grouped them by address, there were six within minutes of her own house. But despite the groupings, the lists all looked the same—the child's name was handwritten in the careful leftward slanting printing Anne Anderson had learned while working years before in the Somerville Public Library. The name was followed by the child's age, address, and the date of diagnosis, the type of leukemia if she knew it, information that had become second nature to Anne. In macabre moments she mentally took what she came to think of as her "leukemia walk," and she imagined herself a tourist guide in her neighborhood, pointing out to visitors "now here on the left is the home of Michael Zona, diagnosed with leukemia on such and such a date, while there on the right is where another boy lives, and here of course is my house." In these moments of almost steeping herself in miserable facts, Anne Anderson would often feel like crying. But she squelched the tears by walking into Jimmy's room because she says, "I knew I wouldn't cry there; I knew I couldn't cry in front of him."

Anne Anderson and Donna Robbins continued comparing notes about the treatment of their sons, and gradually, Donna became aware of Anne's suspicions. "I remember Bruce asking me if I thought there could be a connection and about how our water was." But Donna Robbins did not join Anderson's ranks just yet. She was not herself convinced that her son's leukemia was connected to anything other than plain bad luck.

Robbie continued on his treatment; Jimmy Anderson on his. In 1977 and 1978, two more leukemia cases in children were diagnosed in East Woburn.

In the spring of 1979, Jimmy Anderson remained in the throes of leukemia therapy. He was attending a special school in West Woburn because of his continuing reading problems, but that year he attended classes infrequently because more often than not, he felt too tired or too ill to leave home.

That year too had seen a focusing of national attention on the toxic waste issue, with the matter of Love Canal now squarely on the national plate. Love Canal jogged the memories of Woburn resident Albert Balestieri, who had spent his childhood in Woburn, and in April 1979 he had telephoned the Massachusetts Department of Environmental Quality Engineering (DEQE) to report a rumor he had heard that the Merrimack Chemical Company, which had operated in Woburn from 1863 to 1929, had produced arsenic products. Indeed, until 1914 Merrimack had been a leading producer of arsenic-based insecticides. Balestieri wondered where all the arsenic waste had gone, and Robert Cleary, the young sandy-haired engineer who would ultimately be assigned to monitor events in Woburn closely, made note of Balestieri's call in his log. However, no inspections of the former Merrimack site were made. Balestieri, for his part an active, vocal man who does not generally take "no" for an answer, says he remembered hearing even as a child that chemicals were being dumped in the Woburn area. He did not know of Anne Anderson, nor she of him, and neither did Anderson know of the history of the land around the Industri-Plex Industrial Park. She did not even visit there very much, since she did not do her shopping at the mall adjacent to the site. "It simply wasn't on my route," she says, "mentally or otherwise."

Despite the persistent Woburn odor, which by 1979 was pronounced enough that residents of Reading, the next town, were complaining about it, no official inquiries about what was in the ground around the former chemical production site were ever made. In a sense there was a giant toxic waste dump in view of all, which nevertheless nobody saw.

In May 1979 builders were at work in a scrubby vacant lot abutting the Aberjona River, which flows southwesterly through Woburn. The crew was grading the land to make way for the new Mishawum commuter rail station, which would better link Woburn to Boston's new subway line. While riding their tractors around the lot, some of the builders came up on a collection of 184 55-gallon drum barrels, piled in groups of ten. The men had no idea what the drums might contain, nor did they know that just a mile or so away at Industri-Plex lay enormous pools of toxic waste. However, the workers had heard of midnight dumping, the unscrupulous practice of unsavory waste haulers who, once contracted by a waste producer to haul wastes, instead unload it improperly en route, leaving the headache of real disposal for the person unfortunate enough to come upon the abandoned material.

Partly to get the barrels out of the way of their commuter rail station and partly because they were fearful of continuing to work around the barrels because they did not know if there was a hazard involved, the builders telephoned the Woburn police, who in turn phoned the Massachusetts environmental protection agency, the DEQE. Engineer Richard Chalpin took the call and decided to take a look as well. He knew from experience that midnight dumpers often used a site more than once, and he feared that perhaps not only might the barrels have leaked into the groundwater or the river, but worse, that the dumper might have at some previous time poured wastes straight into the river itself. Since at the time the Aberjona was thought to feed the aquifer on which city wells G and H drew water, Chalpin decided to sample the well water, using the department's recently acquired gas chromatograph mass spectrometer.

Chalpin had not heard of Anne Anderson or the leukemia cases in East Woburn. He had not heard of previous complaints or concern about water quality in wells G and H, and he was not even aware that wells G and H were the main source of water for the East Woburn area. He made the decision to test wells G and H on his own, purely because his awareness of the Love Canal events in specific and the toxic waste problem in general had led him to err in favor of caution. It was a crucial coupling of independent thinking and independent action.

Though the abandoned barrels had contained the chemical polyurethane, the well water did not.

What it did contain, however, set a chain of events

in motion that would shape the turn of events in Woburn and provide Anne Anderson's informal investigation the formal spark it needed. Chalpin's sampling on May 14, 1979, showed that well G contained the following:

Chloroform	11.8 parts per billion (ppb)
Trichloroethylene (TCE)	267.4 ppb
Tetrachloroethylene (PCE)	20.8 ppb
1,1,1-Trichloroethane	0.6 ppb
Dibromochloromethane	2.0 ppb

Well H had no detectable chloroform, trichloroethane, or dibromochloromethane, but it did contain 183.6 ppb of TCE and 13.4 ppb PCE.

The chemicals detected were almost all known carcinogens, although their cancer-causing potential had thus far been observed only in laboratory animals. They were all on an EPA list of hazardous substances, and they were present in the well water in extremely high concentrations. For example, the "risk" level of TCE published by the EPA was 27 ppb, and well G alone contained ten times that amount. Given the results of Chalpin's work, the state of Massachusetts ordered the city of Woburn to shut down wells G and H immediately, which it did on May 22, 1979.

Chloroform was a well-established carcinogen at the time, since data published in 1976 by the National Cancer Institute showed that ingestion of chloroform had caused cancer of the liver in male and female mice, kidney cancers in male rats, and benign thyroid tumors in female rats.

Chloroform is a widely used chemical, both as a fumigant and fungicide for soil, and before the 1976 data was released, humans could come in contact with chloroform whenever it was used as an anesthetic or as a component of cosmetics and toiletries. By 1978 the United States was producing 355 million pounds of chloroform a year, accounting for half the chloroform production in the world, about 2% of which, or 7 million pounds, escaped into the atmosphere as air pollution during the manufacturing process. How much escaped into water was unknown.

Chloroform was found in the private wells near the Toone-Teague road dump in Hardeman County in Tennessee in amounts ranging from 16 to 1,890 ppb. Of course, chloroform can be readily formed during the water chlorination process, and it was the inception of chlorination that made much water fit to drink and rendered many water-borne diseases, such as cholera, obsolete in the developed world. However, chlorination does not usually generate chloroform in extraordinary quantities such as the upper range of the Hardeman County results, or the levels found in wells G and H. According to a study in 1981 by the New Jersey Department of Environmental Protection on toxics in groundwater, levels of chloroform such as those found in Woburn and Hardeman County "undoubtedly occur from direct discharge into the ground."

TCE was present too in unusually high concentrations. An EPA study showed a value of 0.1 to 0.5 ppb to be average in groundwater nationwide, and Woburn had over a thousand times as much.

TCE is a ubiquitous solvent. It easily melts grease from metal, and it is indeed used in almost any industrial process where heavy machinery must be cleaned. It is also used to synthesize and produce other chemicals, as a heat-exchange medium in refrigerators, and as a fumigant, as well as a dry-cleaning agent. TCE was also commonly used to decaffeinate coffee. The chemical is slightly soluble in water, has a low molecular weight, and does not degrade quickly.

A 1976 study by the National Cancer Institute found that TCE, like chloroform, caused liver cancer in mice of both sexes. Rats developed lung tumors, and various malignant tumors of the lymph glands, such as lymphomas and sarcomas, the glands that produce white blood cells, the cells that run amok in leukemia.

On the basis of these studies, in 1979 TCE was considered a definite carcinogen. Even if the chloroform had not been found, the presence of TCE alone would have been enough to force the closing of the wells.

An article in the *Woburn Times* announced the news of the closing of the wells, but by then the Anderson children were preparing for their summer vacation and move to Epping, New Hampshire, where they had rented a cottage. They did not have their Woburn newspaper forwarded to them, and amazingly, with friends scattered here and there for their own vacations, no one let them know about the discovery of the well water contamination.

Consequently, Anne Anderson's main distraction was the rising and falling curve of Jimmy's condition. In general, being in Epping gave him a lift of spirits, perhaps because he had the more frequent company of his brother and sister who did not have to go off each day to school. Sometimes, Jimmy was able to enjoy the outdoors, occasionally taking a swimming lesson, but more often, he sat on the dock watching the other children.

In the evening after supper, Anne Anderson often took walks with other mothers in the twilight lit woods. It was the only time in the day the women saved for themselves, for their children were often out on their own after-supper summer activities, and supper dishes were, at last, all done. But Jimmy, by the end of each day, generally was not up to much, and so often he would accompany his mother and her friends as they strolled around the campground. But just as often he would grow too tired to walk back to the Anderson cottage. On these occasions, he asked his mother to wait with him in the woods until it got darker, so the other children in the camp would not see her carrying him, a thin eleven-year-old boy, home.

The summer of 1979 passed this way for the Andersons, and it was fall again before they learned that G and H wells had been closed and that Patrick Toomey, aged ten, a classmate of Kevin Kane's who had also served as an altar boy with Kevin at St. Joseph's Roman Catholic Church, had received a diagnosis of acute lymphocytic leukemia on August 15 that summer. Innocent of what it meant at first, Patrick said to his parents, "Gee, I'm glad it is not diabetes. That's a really bad disease."

This news was soon compounded.

It seemed that in June, while the Andersons were in Epping, an engineer for the DEQE was driving to work along route 128, passing easily within sight of construction underway at Industri-Plex. His eye caught the glinting construction equipment shoving earth this way and that. He suspected the builders were at work in or near wetlands, those swampy areas protected by the federal

EPA because they were believed to be invaluable components in the ecosystem, fertile nurseries so to speak for insects, birds, and fish. Wetlands are in theory governed by fairly tight zoning regulations, in an attempt to keep them from being paved over by development projects.

In July, EPA investigators inspected the Industri-Plex site to see if the construction was in violation of wetlands zoning regulations. Indeed, the excavation violated federal guidelines, and the United States Army Corp of Engineers issued a "cease and desist" order on June 22 to the Mark Philip Realty Trust, which was developing the site. But the excavators ignored the order, the corps observed when it conducted an aerial inspection of the site several days later. On June 28, excavation finally stopped, and the state level DEQE filed legal papers in an attempt to secure an injunction against the trust to prevent further excavation that could threaten the wetlands.

The pending legal actions sent federal EPA investigators to the site as well, and when they made their inspection, they found more problems than anyone had anticipated.

There, before their eyes on the ground and out of sight below it, were vast pools of toxic waste. One lagoon, 34,918 square feet in area and 5 feet deep, was contaminated with lead and arsenic among other chemicals. Two other pits were located close by, one containing soil contaminated with highly concentrated carcinogenic chromium, the other containing more lead.

But despite the shocking nature of these discoveries and their potential importance, no news was given to the public. And it was not until September 10, when Charles Ryan of the *Woburn Daily Times* broke the story, that the townspeople of Woburn, Anne Anderson and Bruce Young included, learned that the town was the unlucky host of what would later prove to be one of the most extensive and most dangerous toxic waste dumps in the United States. Ryan also reported that no Woburn official had been advised during the summer by the EPA or the DEQE of the discovery. However, later investigations showed that a letter sent in 1972 from the DEQE to the developers of Industri-Plex about the presence of toxic chromium at the site also had a "cc: Woburn Board of Health."

The combination of the well closings and the lagoon discoveries finally made the leukemia cases in East Woburn seem considerably less coincidental to Bruce Young. "Suddenly," he says, "everything Anne had been hammering away at seemed plausible, just from one day to the next."

But Young knew they still needed a firmer sense of the numbers of cases involved and a system better than hearsay. So Young placed an ad in the Woburn newspaper asking anyone who knew of a case of childhood leukemia in Woburn to attend a meeting at the Walker Hall of Trinity Church on October 4.

He and Anne Anderson prepared for the meeting by buying an ordinary quadrant map of Woburn at a local stationery store and by asking John Truman to suggest questions they should pose to any townspeople who might attend. Truman, who had been skeptical of Anne Anderson's theory about a link between the leukemia cases and the water, remained unworried about the prospect of such a link. But he was intrigued enough by the problem since the Industri-Plex waste discovery and the well closings to help in the information-gathering process. He prepared a simple questionnaire.

On October 4, Anne Anderson made a quick dinner for her family and asked Carol Gray to stay with Jimmy while she and Charles Anderson drove over to Walker Hall. Slowly, women and men, mostly couples, began to drift in, and soon there were approximately twenty people. Some were familiar faces—Donna Robbins, Richard and Mary Toomey, Kevin and Patricia Kane, Pat and Joan Zona—as well as some unfamiliar Woburnites neither Anne Anderson nor Young had met before. There had even been families who had kept their child's leukemia to themselves because of fear of stigma.

Anonymity gave way to introductions, and the air was alternately alive with excitement and leadened by sadness, for the business at hand was not joyful, confirmation of leukemia cases among neighbors being, as Anne Anderson puts it, "not exactly something to feel happy about having in common."

Despite their eagerness to tally and plot the results of the meeting, Anne Anderson and Young did not have the chance to do so right away. Anne had to return quickly home after the meeting because Jimmy was feeling especially weak and sick that night. Charles Anderson, for his part, remained unpersuaded that the meeting had turned up something unusual.

Several days later in the Trinity Church office, Bruce Young and Anne Anderson met. There they spread out their simple black and white street map over the files and other papers scattered on Young's desk. Anne took

the questionnaires and called out the addresses and diagnosis dates while Bruce marked the corresponding
spot on the map with a small circle. His marker kept
returning to quadrants G4 and G5 in East Woburn. In
total there were twelve cases, all diagnosed between
1969 and 1979, six tightly grouped near the Anderson
house in what was called the Pine Street area.

A silent look, reflecting more amazement than satisfaction at being right, passed between them. But as
Young says, "we still did not know if twelve was a lot."
He made an appointment with John Truman and went
into Boston to see him. Anne Anderson could not attend
the meeting. Jimmy was feeling too sick that day to leave
with someone else, she felt.

Truman credits the map Bruce and Anne had fashioned with convincing him: "Only when Bruce literally
sat me down and said 'look at this' was the significance
of what Anne had been saying really impressed on my
mind. I picked up the phone and called the Centers for
Disease Control in Atlanta. I think I even did it right
that day."

Fortified by Truman's response, Young then telephoned Charles Ryan at the *Woburn Times,* who wrote
a story on December 12 headlined, "Child Leukemia
Answer Sought." It was the first public recognition of
the cluster, seven years after the private instinct of Anne
Anderson had clicked on. With the involvement of Bruce
Young and John Truman and the potential involvement
of the CDC, the mysterious pocket of leukemia had gone
from being the hunch of a mother with no formal epidemiological training to a riddle that would test the
training of the most experienced epidemiologists in the

country. The Woburn waste dump was no longer just an odiferous nuisance and eyesore. And the illness of an eleven-year-old boy too weak to manage to climb the three front steps of his home now had implications for millions of people.

7

The Presumption of Danger

THE QUESTIONS of what makes a given chemical dangerous to health and of why, how, and when dangerous
chemicals may actually cause human illness are central
to the matter of whether toxic waste sites such as Woburn's are the germs of a modern epidemic of environmentally induced disease. For that the wastes are toxic
and potentially harmful are indisputable facts; more
complicated is the matter of when and how this potential harm is unleashed to manifest itself in humans—
whether in the form of rashes, nervousness, headaches,
dizziness, nausea, birth defects, or cancer. The wish to
avoid disease, rather than the knowledge that suspicious
disease existed in the form of a leukemia cluster, led to
the closings of wells G and H, for that there was a cluster
was not known by those who closed the wells.

In evaluating the impact of toxic waste sites, though
other untoward health effects are also of concern, the
problem of cancer seems to be paramount. Simply put,
a carcinogen is a substance capable of causing cancer,
and in general one learns a substance is capable of causing cancer because it does so. In other words a chemical
might cause a number of effects: it might burn skin; it
might smell; it might take the paint off the hood of a

117

car. But it will not instigate the growth of a cancer unless it is a cancer-causing substance. Carcinogenicity is not an aberrational characteristic that a chemical takes on one day and drops the next. A chemical's inherent ability to cause cancer is constant, and that provides some constancy to the problem of how to evaluate the risks of toxic chemicals. Yet a known, proven carcinogen will not invariably cause cancer in all who cross its path. It is a hit-or-miss proposition as to who will develop a cancer, and a cluster can be thought of as a record of the hits.

The closing of wells G and H was based on a presumption of danger given the presence of known carcinogens in water human beings were using. If the chemicals in question had not been tested for carcinogenicity prior to the time the wells were sampled, the wells might have continued in operation. Therefore how much testing has been done on a given substance determines not only what we know about it, but what we think about its potential impact and what we do about preventing its undesirable effects.

Biologists Dr. Bruce Ames and Dr. Joyce McCann while working at the Berkeley campus of the University of California developed a kind of shorthand test for carcinogenicity called the Ames test in 1973. *Salmonella* bacteria are exposed to the chemical being evaluated to determine whether the genes of the bacteria, whose genetic makeup is not dissimilar to our own, are changed or destroyed. A mutagenic substance, that is, one capable of altering genes, is generally regarded as also being carcinogenic, that is, capable of causing cancer.

The advantages of the Ames test are that it is quick

and cheap, but mainly millions of microscopic bacteria, standing in for humans, can be exposed to the chemical in question in one procedure on a small coaster-size Petri dish. With such a large population of test "subjects," the likelihood of seeing an effect is greater than when only a hundred or so rat or mice subjects are used. This is not to say that in an Ames test the effect is forced; it is simply pushed out into the open by the odds. An effect one might otherwise miss is rendered visible in the way a black felt background might highlight a snowflake. The visibility effect is important, particularly in cluster investigations, because one might not observe disease patterns when only a smallish number of cases are being viewed.

For example, after developing swine flu vaccine, manufacturers tested it on 5,000 human volunteers. Since the volunteers demonstrated no untoward effects, the vaccine was approved, marketed, and administered to 42 million people. Suddenly, untoward effects had more chances to make a "hit," and indeed only amidst this larger background population did the effects show themselves. Two hundred people were paralyzed as a result of the swine flu vaccine. Though this was a fraction of a percent of the total number of people who were given the vaccine, the paralysis is permanent for the "few" people involved, and the effect was worrying enough to lead to a removal of swine flu vaccine from the market.

The Ames test is considered about 90% reliable in determining carcinogenicity, although not for all classes of toxic organic chemicals. However, other tests have been developed so that, in general, whether a chemical is a carcinogen can be established in a laboratory. However, of the roughly 65,000 synthesized chemicals in common use in the United States, virtually nothing is known about the potential health effects of 90% of them, according to an evaluation by the National Academy of Sciences. An Ames test is not performed on chemicals as a matter of course, even though approximately seventy new chemicals are registered for sale each hour in the United States.

Even the carcinogenicity of TCE, one of the chemicals in wells G and H that triggered Chalpin's presumption of danger, had slipped through the Ames test on *Salmonella*, showing no mutagenicity until a metabolite, a breakdown product of TCE called chloral hydrate, was administered to the bacteria. TCE itself, however, did alter the genes in the *Saccharomyces cerevisiae* strain of bacteria, and in 1979 TCE was definitely classified a mutagen.

TCE had also been tested in rats and mice for its potential to induce tumors in tissue. Such tests are sometimes criticized, even ridiculed, by those who have a conservative view of the cancer risk from environmental agents because rats and mice are exposed to high doses of substances compared, quantitatively, to what a human being might encounter in the course of ordinary living. Sometimes one hears such arguments as "a human would have to drink the stuff by the gallon" to reach the equivalent risk of exposure. Certainly one heard that argument when test results revealed that saccharin, commonly added to diet foods and sodas in lieu of sugar, had been shown to be carcinogenic.

In any case, although the transfer from laboratory

animals to humans is unwieldy, it has an important rationale. In the first place there is a moral argument that prevents humans from being subjects in a controlled laboratory experiment with a substance whose effects are unknown. This argument holds, despite our routine use of approved substances about which little is known, which in a sense makes us all test subjects outside the laboratory. In these "tests" the effects may never be known because the "experiment" is informal. No one could morally justify having children inhale asbestos fibers in a laboratory so scientists could see what would happen, but children are allowed to inhale asbestos fiber everyday in schools we know to be insulated with peeling asbestos tiles. Nevertheless we keep the field and the laboratory separate, and use of humans to test carcinogenicity of a substance is certainly frowned upon ethically.

Animals are preferable to humans for practical reasons too, not the least of which is to overcome the latency factor. If animals in test situations are going to develop cancer, they will do it quickly compared to humans whose cancers can develop up to forty years after exposure to a carcinogen. The doses of a chemical to which an animal is exposed are calculated to take this shorter latency into account and are adjusted to allow for differences between rat body weight and human body weight. Also, if anything, humans are more sensitive to toxic effects of chemicals than animals are. Dr. Irving Selikoff's shorthand formula is that humans are 60 times more sensitive than mice, 100 times more sensitive than rats, and 700 times more sensitive than hamsters. Rodents are used, it must be added, because they are cheaper and because the higher on the evolutionary ladder the species, the more likely the public outcry to protect the species. Giving cancer to a rat is not as offensive to public sentiment as giving cancer to an animal one might be likely to have as a pet, such as a cat or dog.

Despite its acknowledged limitations, the laboratory animal test is meant to be a microcosm of the real world. Relatively speaking, a few rodents are exposed to a chemical, and their reactions are then used to predict the effects the chemical might have when millions of people come in contact with it. A typical rodent test for carcinogenicity can involve feeding the animals the chemical, or having them inhale it, observing the condition of a "control" group that is not exposed to the substance or exposed at lower doses, and comparing results.

Of course, the more times a test is done and the same results observed, the more reliable the results. Barring faulty laboratory procedures, such as failing to keep the laboratory animals free of exposure to substances other than the one being tested, a test that turns up more tumors than one would expect to see normally in the rodent population in question generally is enough to establish that the chemical is a carcinogen.

But that is not to say that laboratory tests which do not turn up carcinogenicity totally exonerate a chemical. A negative result could be like the swine flu vaccine: too few animals were tested, or not enough tests were done. And sometimes effects seen in the real world cannot be duplicated by laboratory tests. For example, as of 1984, scientists have not been able to give scrotal cancer to rats by applying soot to their testicles in an attempt to replicate the results observed by Percivall Pott in London among chimney sweeps in 1775. Yet Pott's observations are widely accepted as valid, and the role of tars, believed to have been the culprit in the chimney sweep soot, in causing modern-day lung cancer is quite well established. Benzene, about whose leukemogenic potential in humans there is little debate and doubt in scientific community, has not been associated with leukemia in tests with laboratory animals. This seems to suggest that while animal results may predict effects in humans, humans appear to suffer effects to which animals can be immune or which may take longer in animals to develop than current testing procedures allow.

In theory one could attempt to duplicate the Woburn leukemia cluster in laboratory animals, but thus far no one has tried.

A major problem with such an experiment, however, would be that since one does not know how long wells G and H were contaminated, one does not know how long the contaminants were in the water that reached East Woburn homes. And moreover, since carcinogens were first found only in May 1979, one does not know if at some point prior to the tests there was more carcinogenic contamination.

And there is also the question of how the contaminated water—however and how long it was contaminated—entered the bodies of the children who developed leukemia. Surely they drank it at some times, even those children whose families ultimately switched to bottled water, even the Anderson children who had access to "Nanna's water." Drinking, however, is not the only route by which chemicals in water may enter the body, and it may account for as little as 20% of the amount ingested. Many chemicals are easily inhaled, especially when they are mixed with hot water. In the late 1970s residents of Hardeman County in Tennessee, for example, complained of dizziness or headaches whenever they took showers, unaware not only of the extent of the water contamination but also of the fact that the chemicals that had seeped into their water from the Velsicol dump were being chemically "stripped" from the water molecules by the pressure in the water column and the heat applied to make the shower hot, a process similar to the aeration engineering method that cleans contaminated water by shooting jets of water into the air. The chemicals in the showers were wafting free, their toxicity enhanced with their liberation from the water stream. Jimmy Anderson would have been given at least 1,200 warm baths in the early years of his life, before his diagnosis and certainly before the nature of contamination in wells G and H was known.

And there is the matter of skin absorption. Skin is by definition porous since its mission is to protect the body's tissues while still allowing them to breathe. Toxicology studies have shown that as much as 90% of chemicals ingested by the body enter through the pores of the skin, absorbed by the body's sealing system, and that certain body areas, such as the underarms and genitals, absorb chemicals more readily than others. So a child sitting in a bath has double exposure—inhalation and skin absorption—added to whatever water he or she drinks.

There is also the exposure children may suffer in

utero, for we know that chemicals can cross the placental barrier. The most flagrant example of this was the tragedy of thalidomide in Europe, where mothers who took the approved tranquilizer gave birth to limbless infants. But that these defects were caused by thalidomide had not yet been shown when an application to sell the drug in the United States was made. Only one alert female pharmacologist, Dr. Frances Kelsey, at the United States Food and Drug Administration stood between thalidomide and a license for its approval for use in the United States. She reviewed the European laboratory test data, decided it was scanty on a number of points, requested more details from the company involved, and when the information she received was not to her satisfaction, did not clear the drug for the United States market. When the horrors thalidomide could cause became known and that the United States had been largely spared them by the vigilance of Dr. Kelsey, President John F. Kennedy awarded her a medal.

Another example was the notorious case of diethylstilbestrol (DES), a hormone prescribed to women in the 1940s and 1950s to enhance fertility. In 1971 an alert pediatrician in Boston noticed that some young women whose mothers had taken the drug during pregnancy had developed vaginal cancers. An investigation subsequently revealed that indeed there was a "cluster" of vaginal cancers among daughters of DES-treated mothers.

Given all the possible environmental agents to which Anne Anderson and other mothers in East Woburn were exposed during their lives, including water from wells G and H, it would be extremely difficult, if not impossible, to pinpoint the role of carcinogens ingested during their pregnancies in the development of leukemia in children.

Added to all these variables are the individual variables, the characteristics of each person that may in some way influence the extent to which each is susceptible to a carcinogen. These characteristics are not understood by science at all, except that there is a certain amount of evidence that one can be genetically predisposed to be susceptible to a carcinogen. Whether this predisposition is inherited or acquired is not known. There is also the question of the condition of the body's immunological system, the body processes that fight off viruses and common colds and infections and, one supposes, carcinogens as well. Genetic and individual immunological differences from one person to the next may explain why one person develops cancer and another does not, why one child and not another develops leukemia.

In reality no presently available test methods aimed at attempting to duplicate the Woburn events in a laboratory could possibly take all these variables into account.

Inherent in all tests of chemicals for carcinogenicity is the concept of risk. The word *risk* like *association* is an epidemiological term intended to brush with the concept of *link*. *Risk* is a cousin of the word *cause:* substances may increase the risk of cancer rather than cause cancer. For those who handle the substances or come in contact with them indirectly, the question generally is, how much toxic chemical amounts to how much risk?

Risk calculation is a measure of probability, and it

is contingent somewhat on the concept of "dose response," namely that the more a substance to which one is exposed, the worse its effect, and the higher the risk of experiencing its effects. On the other hand, risk assessment flies in the face of the no-threshold theory, namely, that there is no safe level of a carcinogen and that there is no cancer risk from a carcinogen in question only when there is no exposure to that carcinogen.

As a practical matter, risks are omnipresent in life, but they can be highly theoretical. Driving a car is a favorite example. The population at risk of an automobile accident is all the people who ever travel in an automobile, but we who drive or ride do so without fear because we prefer to think that it is others who are the population at risk, that is to say, not us. The car-traveling public accepts the odds of accidents and the rather high level of risk.

Environmental regulations, also a practical matter, set "safe" standards for a few substances with which the EPA has been able to grapple. According to a report by the Comptroller General of the United States to the Congress published in June 1984, of the 65,000 or so chemicals currently in use, the federal EPA had acted to control only four chemicals, and though it had identified another twenty-two for further testing, it had not finalized the rules under which the chemicals would be tested.

When wells G and H were closed in May 1979, there was no standard for how much TCE could "safely" be in drinking water under the federal Safe Drinking Water Act passed in 1973. There was only knowledge that, as of studies done in 1976, TCE was a carcinogen. So, given that Richard Chalpin did not know about the East Woburn leukemias when he tested wells G and H, it was his own antennae about risk, rather than concrete knowledge of a special nature of risk in Woburn or a particular quantifiable level of risk, that spurred his action.

Later that year on November 26, 1979, in the absence of any "safe" standard for TCE, the Health Effects Branch of the Office of Drinking Water of the EPA issued the flip side of a risk assessment, a SNARL (Suggested No Adverse Response Level), for TCE.

SNARLs are issued to measure short-term effects of a particular substance that might occur as a result of an accident or spill, for example, if a truck filled with TCE were to overturn and break open on a highway, splashing many people, or if a single worker cleaning a printing machine with TCE inadvertently cleaned the rags in the factory drinking water supply. SNARLs do not take into account synergistic effects due to the marriage of the SNARL chemical with other chemicals in the body, or food, or in the open environment. In short, a SNARL is a quick shot at risk assessment intended to provide information about how much exposure one could stand on a one- to ten-day basis before suffering the acute ill effects of toxicity, which for TCE was known to be liver, kidney, and central nervous system damage. SNARLs do not pretend to address the question of long-term risk of cancer from short-term exposures.

Nevertheless, the SNARL calculated in November 1979 on the basis of a child's body weight, when drinking water was presumed to be the principal source of TCE exposure, was 75 micrograms per liter or parts per billion (ppb). When drinking water was presumed to account for only 20% of the potential TCE ingested, the SNARL was set at 15 ppb.

On May 14, 1979, G well contained TCE in the amount of 267.4 ppb, and H well contained 183.6 ppb, so that at least on that one day TCE levels were about three and a half times higher in well G and about two and a half times higher in well H than the SNARL "safe level" if major exposure were to be by drinking. If drinking were not assumed to be the main source of exposure, then G well was approximately eighteen times higher than the SNARL and the H well level was twelve times higher.

Of cancer risk assessment the SNARL for TCE said, "The state of the art at the present time is such that no experimental tools can accurately define the absolute numbers of excess deaths attributable to trichloro-ethylene in drinking water."

One year later, however, a year and a half after wells G and H were closed, in the *Federal Register* the EPA published the methods it used to arrive at some measure of cancer risk for adult humans. The estimates were expressed in terms of the concentration of the chemical in water in parts per billion that if consumed daily over a seventy-year life span would lead to an increased risk of one incidence of cancer per 100,000 people, or one extra cancer case per 100,000 people. For TCE that risk estimate was 27 ppb. That meant that on May 14, 1979, well G contained approximately ten times as much TCE as the risk estimate for adults, and well H contained 6.8 times as much.

The chemicals found at Industri-Plex, such as arsenic and lead, also had their SNARLs and risk estimates, and the amounts found at the site exceeded so called "safe" limits by wide margins. For example, the interim federal standard for arsenic in drinking water in September 1979 when the Industri-Plex lagoons were discovered was 0.05 milligrams per liter, or parts per million (ppm), but in one pit alone, arsenic was concentrated as high as 1,100 ppm. Since very little arsenic was found in wells G and H in May 1979, but TCE, which had not been found at Industri-Plex, was present in large amounts, it became clear that the way water circulated underground in Woburn would have to be determined if the potential health effects of the toxic wastes in Woburn could be calculated and the level of overall contamination evaluated.

This was one prong of official activity, but in the late fall of 1979, neither Anne Anderson, nor Bruce Young, nor any of the other parents, were being talked to by officials about SNARLs or risk estimates or whether indeed there could be a link between toxics in the soil and water and the leukemia cluster. For one thing, even that there was a bona fide cluster remained to be officially verified. The homemade G4-G5 quadrant map compiled in Bruce Young's office looked dramatic, but it would require further study.

In January of 1980 Bruce Young, Donna Robbins, and Anne Anderson, together with a group of about twenty other Woburn residents, some of whom were parents of children with leukemia or friends of the cluster families, formed an organization they hoped could coordinate information about toxic waste and health in Woburn and share it with the public at large. They called the group FACE (For a Cleaner Environment) and began issuing a simple newsletter called *FACE Facts*.

In the meantime the Centers for Disease Control (CDC) in Atlanta, Georgia, began evaluating the call it received from John Truman about the incidence of leukemia in East Woburn. Established as the Communicable Disease Center in 1946, the CDC had grown from the nucleus of an agency called Malaria Control in War Areas (MCWA). The centers' main mission was to track and prevent infectious diseases. In the wake of Love Canal the CDC was slowly being drawn into an entirely new area of epidemiology, one in which the agents were not rare germs but chemicals people used in their daily lives. John Truman's call came at a time when the centers' cancer branch was receiving similar calls from citizens suspecting cancer clusters at the approximate rate of one a day.

The toxic waste problem thrust the CDC out of its traditional role as the monitor of infectious disease and into the territory of such institutions as the National Cancer Institute and the National Institute of Occupational Safety and Health. Yet the CDC, the venerable institution of the study of epidemics, had a history of experience on which to draw in order to attempt to lasso the elusive answer to the basic question: was the Woburn cluster a mini-epidemic with a particular cause or not?

In this new CDC territory of numerous potential environmental causes related to pollution and contamination, there was also impressive new technology and new methods for tracking the villains down. The measurement techniques were more precise than anything even imagined when the Panama Canal was being built or when the CDC was being established. The presence of villians could be detected to the most minute amount.

It was no longer a matter of using the naked eye to see if there were mosquito beds in the swamp or whether there was a particular germ under the microscope. The cause of the epidemic now might be an invisible quantity of a chemical whose actual mechanism for causing disease was poorly understood. For the CDC, tracking environmental culprits in the 1980s was as challenging a business as searching for the causes of tropical diseases in the 1900s. Although in some ways there were many more tools, there was not always enough information about how to use them.

Dr. John Cutler, a CDC staff epidemiologist with a long, narrow face and a salt-and-pepper beard, who was eventually assigned to design and administer the Woburn cluster investigation, commented on the femtomole, for example, the amount of toxic material capable of invading the genetic material of a single cell. Impressed with the power of that technology on the one hand, but skeptical of its practical implications on the other, Cutler commented, "I don't know what we can do with a measurement like that except scare people."

Toxic Tinkering

THE HUMAN BODY contains as many as 75 trillion cells, each capable of metabolizing substances to produce energy and of reproducing so that various organs can develop and be maintained. The cell is the basic unit of independent life, the smallest coin in the currency of the human body.

Cells are constantly dying and replacing themselves. There are an average of 25 trillion red blood cells in the body at any given time, and each one lives about four months. Other cells last less long, and the endless process of cell replacement takes place in the body at the virtually inestimable speed of 10 million cells a second.

Every new cell comes with a set of genetic operating instructions, so to speak, which tells the cell what to do. This information, what is often called the genetic code, determines our sex, the color of our eyes, our looks, the basic capabilities of our minds. And it may ultimately determine whether we will be well or not.

It is the cells, not the scientists, that hold the answers. And in a cluster like Woburn's, although epidemiology involving questionnaires and paperwork and statistical analyses seem distant from the human cell, answers to the question of what may have caused a mysterious cluster lie with learning whether some intrusion on the cell, as well as some misprinting or misreading of the genetic instructions, caused the cancers in question.

This learning does not come in giant bites, but rather in the incremental acquisition of information that is the style of the scientific method. And though the general public, especially the post–World War II generation, tends to view science as a source of answers, scientists would probably say their goal is the gathering of information based on the systematic exploration of theories. One is a flash, the other a constant flicker. The public expectation is fed in part by public admiration of the long years of academic study and field training that shape a scientist and the density of the things that scientists sometimes say. As Anne Anderson observed, "we are raised to think of scientists as a group apart from us, that they are the ones who really know things."

Too there is curiosity about science, evidenced by the proliferation in the early 1980s of popular science magazines and television programs. They reduced the painstaking time-consuming nature of proper research to episodes and perhaps made it seem science moves faster than it actually does. Most likely the breadth of disciplines like biology and epidemiology and toxicology, let alone of the super subspecialty sciences like molecular biology and cytotoxicology, is not generally appreciated by the public.

Nor does the average person have a daily need to know about the interdependence of these sciences, the building block nature of basic research that puts each investigation in relationship to what came before with scientists following each other's leads—repeating experiments, refuting and supporting each other, disclaiming, proclaiming, and exclaiming. Scientists generally have a polite way of roaring at each other, but roar they do nevertheless.

The science of cancer—its causes and its cures—is full of roaring. And it may be especially volatile precisely because it crosses the boundaries of many disciplines. Any scientist thinking about what causes cancer is, by definition, thinking about the essential question of what makes life go haywire, and this means looking through many lenses at the same object: the human cell.

Every normal human cell except germ cells, which determine sex, is governed by a set of chromosomes, 46 in all, arranged in 23 pairs, one of each pair from each parent. The chromosomes ride the genes, carrying the information the cell needs to start its business, which is to say its life. The information is a blueprint, so to speak, for the development of cellular chemicals, for example, enzymes and proteins, the substances that fuel cell metabolism and therefore life.

Genes, of which there are 50,000 to 100,000 in each of us, are composed of nucleic acids, chained in ways that have been compared to words in a sentence. As the choice and arrangement of words determine what a sentence says, the choice by the genes of what proteins and enzymes to order the cell to make determines the business of each cell and thus the business of the body.

Of the nucleic substances, the most important is deoxyribonucleic acid (DNA), a macromolecule that is the fundamental substance of the gene, the library of cellular information.

The search to determine what DNA looked like and

how it worked was a pointed example of how even the greatest of scientific revolutions are evolutionary in nature. That life proceeded through heredity, one generation to the next, was suggested by the Austrian monk and botanist Gregor Mendel in 1865. However, his ideas went largely unaccepted until the turn of the twentieth century. After that the study of human genetics still remained abstract, with scientists busy working on plants and fruit flies. Only in the 1930s and 1940s with the development of biochemistry did it become known that human genes were in fact composed of nucleic acids. In 1944 Dr. Oswald Avery of the Rockefeller University discovered that it was DNA which transmitted the genetic information chemically. But how this was accomplished would remain a mystery until the structure of DNA could be known.

James D. Watson and Francis Crick cracked this problem in 1953, showing the world that DNA was designed in twin spiral strands, joined by chemical cross links and bars like the steps of an elegant spiral staircase. Watson's book *The Double Helix* details the search to describe this fine design, which is the switching system of all life.

But also in Watson's book are descriptions of the "roar" of the science that rumbled along the trail of discovery. In those days Dr. Linus Pauling, for example, the eminent Nobel Prize–winning biochemist, had aroused the ire of his colleagues by what some thought of as melodrama. For example, at the time Pauling was in hot pursuit of how proteins were constructed, and when he had at last determined the structure, he built a model of it. When he announced his findings to the scientific world, he kept the model behind a curtain while he talked. Then, like a bride to suitors who had missed their chance to marry her, Pauling unveiled the model.

There was, according to Watson, some applause and some murmurs: "There was no one like Linus in all the world. The combination of his prodigious mind and his infectious grin was unbeatable. Several fellow professors, however, watched his performance with mixed feelings. . . . If only he had shown a little humility, it would have been so much easier to take! . . . A number of his colleagues quietly waited for the day when he would fall flat on his face by botching something important."

Biochemistry was a new field at the time, and it was full of opposing conceptual camps and varying competencies. Watson confides that at a crucial point in their DNA research, he and his colleague Crick were taken off the project by their superior principally because he did not understand the significance of what they were doing. But they persisted, and aided by the developing technology of x-ray crystallography, which enabled them to have outline pictures of the DNA molecule, they came up with a structure that made both chemical and structural sense, given the crystallographs.

Pauling too had been hoping to find the structure of DNA, but Crick and Watson did it first, and Watson described Pauling's concession they had won as "graceful." The thin double strand made sense, and as Watson put it, a "structure so beautiful had to be right."

A structure so beautiful was also very very important.

Four basic nucleic acids strung together in two chains

make up a DNA molecule—guanine and adenine on one side, and cytosine and thymine on the other. In stable basic DNA the two strands are complementary and entwined. Adenine always pairs with its opposite, thymine; and guanine always pairs with cytosine. When cells divide, the offspring cell contains DNA identical to that in the parent cell. To put some of itself into the new cell, to replicate, the DNA spiral molecule unwinds, each single strand now capable of synthesizing a new double strand, a new double helix. Each new helix in each new cell goes on with the task at hand, having inherited the four basic acids of DNA. These four can order up, or "code for," all the other substances—enzymes, proteins, and so forth—the body needs, depending on the task at hand. Thus, like a do-it-yourself artisan, the replicating DNA molecule assembles the chemicals, and through the intermediary acid, the messenger RNA (ribonucleic acid), the DNA gets the orders out from the cell nucleus and into the cytoplasm, where metabolism takes place. The amount of DNA in one single cell is enough to code for 1 million different acid chains that make up the biochemicals used in cell metabolism.

Cell reproduction is tightly controlled by this DNA-dictated biochemistry.

For it is the subtle changes in the combination of the chemicals that tell a cell whether it will be a skin cell, a blood cell, liver cell, brain cell, and so forth. It is this perfectly orchestrated chemical process that programs a fertilized egg to develop into a fetus and ultimately a baby complete with all necessary parts. In theory, a fouled-up DNA molecule could program itself to turn out a body made only of liver cells or only of brain cells.

Such a body could not work, but in theory it could be made. However, a healthy genetic system turns out all the infinitely distinct cells of the body's different organs. The creation and replacement of cells, appropriately, accounts for the astounding miracle of life. The out-of-control proliferation of cells is the renegade we call cancer.

It is obviously true that the body itself is composed of chemicals. And in discussing the possible role of environmental hazards in the development of cancer, one tends to talk of chemicals as if they were factors in the environmental hazards external to the body, an insult from outside it. Clearly it is a complex interaction of chemicals—external and internal—that is involved in causing cancer.

A carcinogenic chemical can act as an initiator of cancer, which means it may start the cell on the road to wrongness. How likely a carcinogen is to act depends on how much carcinogen is on the scene. One single exposure to a carcinogen, depending on its potency, can be enough to at least initiate carcinogensis, and it is generally accepted that there is no level of exposure considered "safe."

In the Woburn context the question arises did something in wells G and H enter the DNA workshop, causing it to code for wrong substances and wrong cells, leukemic cells, instead of right ones?

The mechanism whereby a cell is initiated to become cancerous could have much to do with DNA. How a cell metabolizes or reacts chemically to an entering carcinogen relates to tumor initiation and the process called covalent binding, where a foreign substance makes itself at home in the DNA molecule, changing the DNA itself or the orders it places for other chemicals.

Carcinogens can literally bind to the DNA like glue, sticking on a step of the spiral stairs. These modified steps are called adducts, and their presence could change the template of the DNA so that when it next unwinds, the next time it reproduces, it has a new plan to follow. The adduct has set new goals for the offspring cell.

A cell initiated with new orders is then ripe to carry them out, ready for the "promotion" stage. In this second phase the initiated or primed-to-go-wrong cell may suffer additional exposure to the original carcinogen. Or a totally different carcinogenic substance may appear and act synergistically to move the process along. A promoter substance alone cannot cause cancer, but initiating substances may also promote, thus doing double duty as agents of cellular change. As to which substances are promoters, which are initiators, and which can be both, science is almost totally in the dark.

A cell carrying incorrect instructions from the DNA, initiated and primed, may well become carcinogenic. And since the bad instructions have been institutionalized, so to speak, in the DNA molecule, every time the cell reproduces, it will do so according to the substituted incorrect plan. It has become an outlaw, a delinquent, living separate from the rules that govern the behavior of the other cells. Fetal cells, at work developing into an entirely new body, newborn tissue, and regenerating wounded tissue, are particularly vulnerable to the error because DNA is extra busy synthesizing itself to meet the demand for cells. There are simply more numerical chances for error.

It was long generally believed that cancer is of monoclonal origin, that is, that a cancer begins in one single cell that duplicates itself over and over again. This would mean that the incorrect brew of enzymes and proteins, generated by the DNA, would generate genetically identical cancer cells, all going the same wrong way. However, research in July of 1984 by a group of scientists at Stanford University found that B-cell lymphoma, a type of cancer of the lymph nodes, could be biclonal, that is, developing from two separate cells of different genetic origin. Again, which cancers are biclonal and which monoclonal is baffling to scientists.

The idea that external chemicals could enter a cell and bind to the DNA found real possibility as an area of research only since the mid-1970s with the advent of the gas chromatograph mass spectrometer, an extremely sophisticated piece of equipment that enables scientists to identify and "mark" minute amounts of chemicals to follow their metabolic paths inside cells. It is this same piece of equipment that made it possible to detect the minute levels of carcinogens present in well G and H water in 1979.

The metabolic process within the body is the key to understanding how carcinogenic substances act in the body. Metabolism is the process wherein the body comes to terms with the myriad substances inside it. The digestive system, for example, metabolizes food, breaking a steak down into a slurry of proteins the body can absorb. At the cellular level the metabolism is even more profound. Through metabolism the body nourishes each and every tiny corner, and also through metabolism the body eliminates useless or poisonous substances. For example, the kidneys keep metabolizing substances until they at last produce a metabolite soluble in water that can be excreted as urine. The liver too is crucial to the detoxification of substances, metabolizing and filtering all the time. But not every substance that comes through the system can be processed and rendered harmless. Metabolic overload also has a lot to do with carcinogenesis, again depending specifically on the chemical in question.

One fairly well-studied chemical has been benzopyrene, a carcinogen found in tobacco smoke, ambient air pollution due to the burning of fossil fuels, and barbecue fumes, among other things. It was observed by several scientific investigators that benzopyrene, metabolized in a cell, broke into different forms, including one with the rather intimidating lengthy label 7B,8a-dihydroxy-9a10a-epoxy,7,8,9,10-tetrahydrobenzopyrene. The name itself is its diagram, describing the chemical structure of the metabolite form, each number referring to its position on the honeycomb, hexagonally shaped carbon rings and appendages that form organic chemicals.

This metabolite or epoxy-adduct form can literally glue itself, like any epoxy would, to one of the DNA steps, namely at the 2-amino position of the acid guanine, what is called the minor groove of the double helix, according to research by Dr. I. B. Weinstein of the Columbia University School of Public Health. Some cells confronted with the original benzopyrene may make a vain attempt to get rid of it, metabolizing it into the epoxy form, which in turn adheres to the DNA, where it becomes a permanent fixture with the potential to set into motion the hierarchy of initiation and promotion and the ensuing series of carcinogenic events.

Sometimes enzymes in a cell can excise the adduct, loosening it and sliding it away somewhat like a label slides off a wine bottle steeped in hot water. But sometimes the cell cannot repair the DNA damage, and the adduct literally sticks around, ready to seize the opportunity to do harm.

Finding adducts and seeing them is a fascinating new area of genetic biology but one that means working in an infinitesimally small universe. An adduct can be formed by a femtomolic amount of a substance, a femtomole being a million billionths or 10^{-15} of a mole. Moles or gram molecules are a measure of the atomic weight of a substance. A femtomole of salt equals roughly a million billionths or 1 quadrillionth of 4 tablespoons. A femtomole of water is roughly equivalent to a million billionths of a cubic inch of water.

To locate such tiny amounts within the DNA molecule, scientists resort to a rather ingenious system that mimics the way the cells fight off disease. Foreign substances, or antigens, such as germs, stimulate the creation of antibodies uniquely suited to seek out, isolate, and vanquish the invader. To find out if there are benzopyrene adducts, antigens, hiding in the DNA, one must create an antibody that will go out and look for them.

To make the antibody, usually the first step is to inject the antigen, the benzopyrene metabolite epoxy form, into a rabbit or other animal. The animal then naturally produces the antibody necessary to fight the antigen off. This antibody substance is then withdrawn from the animal and can be used to "probe" cells in which one is looking for adducts. Once injected into a cell, the antibody will automatically seek its adversary, like a heat-seeking missile, leading the scientist straight to the antigen—the adduct—if there is any to be found. Antibodies have only one target; they will hunt out only the particular antigen for which they were formed. Therefore this is a rather effective method for finding out where chemical intruders might be lodging in the grooves of the DNA.

But the method is no simple matter. Just producing enough of the antibody, for example, can take months. And matching antibodies have been synthesized for very few antigenic substances. There is as of this writing, for example, no antibody available to seek out TCE adducts, and it would take a full-time, first-rate team working with unlimited funds at least six months to come close to developing one.

The world of adduct research is one of strict precision. In the spring of 1985, Dr. Regina Santella, working with Dr. Weinstein's research group at Columbia University, was overseeing the biochemistry of some adduct studies. The work requires painstaking chemical theorizing and a steady hand.

At first glance the adduct laboratory looks simple—vials and beakers and the traditional sound of clinking glassware familiar to all who took a high school chemistry course. There are also simple plastic trays, each indented with ninety-six half-bubbles about as wide as a No. 2 pencil and as deep as its eraser. Into these tiny depressions, scientists gently pipette 200 nanograms of DNA, a submicroscopic quantity, which is ultimately analyzed in an ordinary looking machine smaller than a typewriter that reads fluorescence and costs about $12,000.

Looking for adducts usually begins with taking a sample of human blood or placental fluid, spinning it down in a centrifuge to separate whole cells from liquid plasma, scraping off the buffy layer of red cells, and extracting DNA from the white cell layer. Then the scientists introduce the yellow-green antibody they have developed to the antigen or adduct form of benzopyrene. Eureka smoke does not rise.

In this procedure the absence of color—a plastic tray of half-bubbles that looks empty but is not—means a positive result. For if there are benzopyrene adducts present in the DNA from the blood sample, the yellowish antibody has found its target, penetrating into the DNA and "disappearing" as far as the naked eye is concerned into the solution. On the other hand, if there is no target adduct for the antibody to ferret out, the antibody will simply stick to cups of the tray, turning it yellow, or stay visible in solution. Of course, there are degrees of reaction: the less color left behind, the more DNA adducts in the sample, and the shades of yellowishness are read as fluorescence in the $12,000 machine.

But, so what if the DNA is full of adducts?

Must an altered DNA molecule necessarily cause a cancer? Do the adducts actually do harm? In theory all of us may have benzopyrene adducts in our DNA because we all breathe in some amount of benzopyrene. Yet fortunately we all do not have cancer of the lung.

So the key element of adduct research involves not only determining how prevalent the DNA adducts are, but whether their presence has any relationship to the presence of cancer. Such research forms the new science of molecular epidemiology.

Dr. Frederica Perera, also in Dr. Weinstein's laboratory at the Columbia University School of Public Health, supervised the epidemiological aspects of a study of benzopyrene adducts scheduled to run into 1986. Using tissue and blood samples from volunteer lung cancer patients and a control group, the team hopes to learn the condition of the DNA in lung cancer patients, in lung tumor cells, and ultimately to learn whether there is any relationship between the level of adduct damage and smoking.

The study sought to distinguish between heavy smokers, light smokers, and nonsmokers. Like traditional epidemiological studies, it began with a questionnaire that collected information about the patient's smoking habits, diet, and other life-style factors. Then blood samples were screened for the presence of the benzopyrene adduct on the hypothesis that if the adduct played a role in causing lung cancer, the lung cancer patient would exhibit more presence of adduct. And if smoking contributed to the formation of benzopyrene adducts, then heavy smokers in theory would exhibit more benzopyrene adducts than light smokers and nonsmokers.

A similar study was also undertaken by the National Institutes of Health in which placental fluid samples were taken from volunteer pregnant women—smokers, nonsmokers, and controls—in an attempt to determine whether a mother who smoked could contribute to adduct formation in a child.

Of course such studies have a major flaw: they are conducted after a cancer has formed in a patient and after the event or events that may have caused the cancer are over. And while much can still be learned, since a tumor in progress in theory is being fueled by renegade DNA, the ideal way to do such a study would be while exposure to the causative carcinogen was still taking place.

Largely because some funding for the adduct studies came from the Council for Research on Tobacco and because the association between smoking and lung cancer is strong, benzopyrene was singled out as a carcinogen to study because it is a known component of tobacco smoke.

There would be no comparable way to investigate the working of TCE, the prime chemical in question at Woburn, until there was an antibody to the metabolites of TCE. Nor, for the same reason, could benzene, the most commonly accepted chemical leukemogen, be investigated in 1985. Therefore, in order to be directly relevant to Woburn, adduct research would have to focus on the chemicals and diseases found there.

In the late 1980s and 1990s another of the most active areas in cancer research will likely be the investigation of cellular oncogenes, genes that are part of normal cells which have the potential to determine whether a cell will become cancerous, and proto-oncogenes, the oncogene's precursor. Both types are essentially normal genes, but somehow they program themselves to set a series of events in motion at the level of a single cell beginning the runaway process of cancer. By mid-1985, approximately twenty different oncogenes linked to different cancers or stages of cancer had been identified, but still remarkably little was known about how they worked. What seemed to be generally accepted was that the genes are not "on" all the time, that they switch themselves on and off. They seemed to be highly active, for example, during times when cells must work furiously, say, during an embryonic stage, which would be consistent with the requirements of high growth also needed to make a tumor.

What turns the oncogenes on is biochemical, and perhaps instead of coding for or ordering the protein needed for normal growth, the oncogene switches the order to a chemical that might spur a tumor. Since DNA is the substance in the gene responsible for ordering, a fault in the DNA mechanism could be linked to the activating of oncogenes. Consequently it is theoretically possible that an adduct in DNA could be what trips the initial wrong message, which the cell cannot call back, and a normal gene becomes oncogenic. In theory as part of the initiating state of cancer growth an adduct may be a part of the activation of a gene's cancerous potential, or a reactivation once the oncogene has shut itself down. In this the adduct could be like one faulty measurement made in a complicated design for a dam. The mistake may go forever unnoticed; fail-safe systems in the inherent design may prevent the mistake from ever causing harm. But then again, a combination of events may compound the measurement error and finally cause the dam to burst. On the other hand, adducts may have nothing whatsoever to do with oncogenes. They may be two entirely separate cellular phenomena, each playing independent perhaps mutually exclusive roles in cellular activity and cancer development.

Cellular changes involved in cancer need not begin within the cell nucleus and DNA alone. According to a chapter in the 1985 edition of *Cecil Textbook of Medicine*,

"The growth of cells is regulated by an interdigitating network that spans from the surface of the plasma membrane to the depths of the nucleus. If that network were to be touched at any point by an adverse influence and tilted out of balance, cancerous growth might ensue."

Another frontier of molecular epidemiology, then, might well be the very frontier of the cell, or the cell receptor, proteins found on the surface of a cell. These receptors appear to be the "lock" on the cell, opened only by a very specific chemical "key." For example, it was suggested by a team of researchers in February 1985 that perhaps in the severest forms of diabetes it is the failure of cell receptors to insulin—locks being approached with wrong keys—which makes some diabetic patients resistant to insulin treatment. In such cases, only large doses of insulin can offset the body's failure to produce its own, which is the cause of diabetes. The insulin receptor protein consists of 1,370 amino acids arranged in an exact order, a highly specific "key."

Adducts, that is, DNA damage, may also play a role in confusing the cell's receptor mechanism and the fit of the lock to the key. In theory, fouled DNA molecules could order mutated proteins and enzymes for the surface of the cell, disrupting the lock system that governs what comes in and out, allowing substances into the nucleus which should not be there—carcinogens. This role for DNA, though highly speculative, is plausible.

The region between a cell's nucleus and its skin was greatly illuminated by Dr. William DeDuve, head of the International Institute of Cellular and Molecular Pathology in Brussels, as well as the Department of Biochemical Cytology at the Rockefeller University. In 1974 he won the Nobel Prize for his discovery of the lysosome, a particle within the cell membrane but outside the nucleus, which functions as the cell's stomach. He also perceived the importance of lysosomes in cancer treatment because a successful treatment is one that kills only the cancerous cells and does not destroy healthy cells by overwhelming the cell's digestive system. The potent drugs of cancer chemotherapy can overpower the lysosomal system for detoxifying substances not meant to be inside the cell.

Studying this system in the lysosomes could also provide some interesting if theoretical clues to how exposure to ambient toxic substances, like those in air or groundwater, might affect the body. For example, it was known that drugs given to prevent malaria, like drugs given to treat cancer, could also seriously damage the liver as a side effect. The liver, the most important detoxifying organ in the body, gets busy to neutralize the toxic agent, the malaria drug, and is damaged in the process. DeDuve's research suggested that this damage took the form of harming the lysosomes in the liver, breaking their own protective membrane and causing them to release their digestive enzymes into the cell, a problem analogous to the overloading of the oil filter on an automobile. The liver may enlarge, because of the release of these substances, in an attempt to keep working, although its filtering capacity has long since been overcome.

Carcinogenic chemicals too pass through the liver system and may do the liver damage, perhaps by damaging its lysosomes, even if there is no cancer in the body. Indeed liver damage is a symptom of exposure to chemicals of which the body is attempting to rid itself. First-round liver damage can take the form of an enlarged liver and can be an indicator of an overtaxed filtering system, leaving one susceptible to a second round of assault by carcinogens or other toxic substances. So enlarged livers or abnormal liver function tests found in residents of, for example, Toone-Teague Road in Hardeman County, Tennessee, in fact may have reflected damage to the lysosomes due to exposure to contaminated water.

The existence of lysosomes was speculated upon long before their discovery, according to Dr. DeDuve. In a talk he gave in 1984 at the Mary Imogene Bassett Hospital in Cooperstown, New York, affiliated with Columbia University, he pointed out that Rudolf Virchow, the founder of the study of pathology, conceptualized lysosomes in a drawing he made in 1857. But Virchow's theories about the pathological breakdown of cells were all but discredited about twenty-five years later when Pasteur and Koch discovered microbes and advanced the theory that it was these tiny organisms that caused disease. It became an either-or scientific battle: if diseases were caused by infectious agents, then they could not be caused by sick cells, and scientists, intoxicated by the discovery of the microbial world, virtually ignored Virchow's ideas.

It was for DeDuve, more than a century later, to reinstate their validity and to expound their implications.

In our time, most of what is suspected about alterations in cell mechanism, particularly the role of DNA and cancer, is highly theoretical. One can draw a cell, and the theoretical process. Like the atomic chain reaction prior to Einstein, the cellular reaction can be suggested, but its precise mechanism is a solar system away from being understood.

These theoretical genetic theories are not without their detractors, who form the basis of another either-or debate about the relationship between cell function and cancer. The epigenetic theory of cancer growth suggests that malignancy may not start at home at all, that is, at the very basis of the cell in its genetic makeup, and that the event which causes cancer is not a mutational mistake which cannot be reversed. Epigeneticists argue that since some kinds of tumors do remit naturally, that is stop growing, the delinquency of tumor cells is reversible and therefore cannot be genetically fixed.

So the submicroscopic environment of the cell is not only a scientific technical frontier, but grounds for an intellectual ferment not unlike the eighteenth century argument over whether disease was caused by living a life of sin, and the nineteenth century battle over whether it was germs or the degeneration of cells to watch out for.

Some of the most fascinating advances in understanding the possible role of cell-level changes in the development of cancer came more than a decade after Jimmy Anderson's diagnosis. And while the full meaning of those advances could be debated, they do present some provocative ideas.

If, for example, Anne Anderson's earliest suspicions had led to an investigation and some of the advanced technology had been available, blood and tissue samples might have been taken from the leukemic children be-

fore they started chemotherapy and examined specifically for DNA and other genetic damage or stored for
future examination. The samples would have covered at
least the years between 1972 when Jimmy was diagnosed and 1979 when the wells were shut down. Had
the blood of the children shown TCE adducts, for example, and the wells were later found to have contained
high amounts of TCE, there would have been useful and
convincing evidence that the wells had been implicated
in causing the unusual leukemia incidence. Liver cells
might also have been examined to see if the body's detoxification mechanism had been attacked.

But in the 1970s, gas chromatography and the mass
spectrometer were not generally available to scientists:
the science of adducts was practically unknown, as was
the idea of examining DNA using adduct antibodies;
lock-and-key receptor theory was undeveloped; few had
heard of lysosomes; and practically no one was listening
to Anne Anderson.

9

The Death of a Child

WITH THE NEWS broken that there was an enormous toxic waste site in Woburn and the suspicion that there was a cluster, if yet unverified, of leukemia, events began to overtake the city.

It became clear that town officials had little experience handling such environmental problems and certainly no idea how to dispose of such massive wastes. In fact, apparently unaware of the possibility that toxic wastes could seep underground, the city engineer, Thomas Mernin, suggested to the press that the town might cover the chemical lagoons with several feet of earth and then pave them over to use them as parking lots. The mounds of chemical hides, he added, could be covered again with earth and then planted with grass.

Tension between bodies of city government erupted, with various units, like the local board of health, complaining they had not been informed about the toxic waste situation and its implications for public health. Charles Ryan, however, of the *Woburn Daily Times*, continued his aggressive reporting on the subject and published his story that, on the contrary, the board of health had received a copy of a letter that the Massachusetts Department of Environmental Quality Engineering (DEQE) had sent to the D'Annolfo development firm engineers working at Industri-Plex as early as 1972, confirming then the presence of toxic chromium, at least, on the property. But no attempt by the city to look into the matter was made. And one wonders, on the other hand, if a mere "cc: Board of Health" copy sent to no individual by name, was an effective way for a state agency to inform a municipality of a potentially dangerous situation.

The media attention Woburn drew as a result of the discovery of the waste site and the leukemia cluster displeased some local officials. When on December 19, 1979, the Woburn City Council met to formally ask the Centers for Disease Control to look into the Woburn health situation, City Alderman Paul Meany said, before the vote, "the publicity has not shed good light on Woburn." Woburn's mayor, then Thomas M. Higgins, also laced into the media, and obliquely Anne Anderson and Bruce Young, saying the day after the city council vote, "the city is not in business for publicity purposes or guess work when it comes to the health and safety of the public, and for anyone with little or no authority to give the impression that there is a major health problem within the confines of the city without factual evidence to back their statements is totally irresponsible."

Momentum for shooting the messenger of bad news was beginning to build, but little was being done to address the bad news itself. Indeed, Anderson and others saw the very agencies charged with helping them in apparent disarray. On Christmas Eve, 1979, the Massachusetts Department of Public Health released a study that seemed to contradict the homemade map Anderson and Bruce Young had compiled. The department said it had uncovered eighteen leukemia deaths, when 10.9 were expected, and that that was not unusually high for a ten-year period. The department also found there did not appear to be a strong pattern of clustering or geographical grouping of deaths. This report was soon proved incorrect.

As events began to unfold in Woburn, at no time were the members of For a Cleaner Environment (FACE), Bruce Young and Anne Anderson in particular, directly contacted by any official of their town or local government with an offer of support or an expression of concern. It was as though what Young and Anderson had found and what had been found in Industri-Plex were grand illusions, which if ignored would go away. And consequently, FACE members lost faith in the ability of their local government to take the situation in hand.

Speaking retrospectively, Representative Nicholas Paleologos, a life-long Woburn resident who had become one of the youngest members of the Massachusetts State Legislature in 1977, analyzed the atmosphere at the time. "Here was a chance for local government to step in and show its citizens it cared. But instead it stonewalled. It saw the situation as a giant public relations nightmare. It was like the officials involved went to the costume closet and passed up the hero's outfit and said 'give me that villain suit—I want to put that one on.' In wanting to keep everything cool, they actually chose the villain's role." FACE decided to go as high as it could and contacted the office of Senator Edward M. Kennedy, and a Kennedy representative visited Woburn to hear about the information the community had collected about leukemia in Woburn.

But, on balance, Anne Anderson felt what she and Bruce had established was going largely ignored. Her clock ran faster than that of the institutions responsible for looking into the evidence she had found. Her time-table was set by the fact that she faced the reality of the leukemia cluster every day in Jimmy's illness.

"That it was taking so long for people to take what we were saying seriously began eating at me," she re-members. But when Bruce Young and two other mem-bers of FACE asked for a meeting with the mayor of Woburn in early 1980, Anne Anderson did not attend for a number of reasons.

Her life still revolved around her home and in par-ticular around Jimmy's condition, which was at that point extremely unpredictable. He was still on chemo-therapy, Dr. John Truman having tailored a standard treatment protocol to Jimmy Anderson's particular case. But the potent treatments exhausted him and often made him sick. He was now nearly twelve years old, but he was almost always out of school because he needed comfort or medical attention or just plain distraction from the routine of feeling lousy. Since he was at home so much during the days, he and his mother became almost inseparable.

She watched him adjust to a life of quiet play at home—running matchbox cars up and down the living room carpet or converging favorite trucks on a make-shift garage. He built endless constructions of Legos plastic bricks or Lincoln logs. His days were often sol-itary, for since he was missing a good deal of school, he did not have a regular group of playmates and the nor-mal after-school routine. And he was sometimes taunted on the rare occasions when he was well enough to play outside. Wearing a baseball cap to cover his thin hair, he was nevertheless called "Baldie" by some tough boys who hoped to make him cry. And if he did not, the boys might actually tear the cap from his head so that Jimmy was too embarrassed to stay outside. Now and then he would relate these episodes to his family, and his older brother, Chuck, would get into brawls with the boys who had been tormenting Jimmy. But mostly, Jimmy developed his own brand of living, a coping at-home style, which was also largely uncomplaining, and fed by a quiet courage. According to his mother, "It was as though he was always bracing himself inside for whatever might be next to come." Faced with the constant stress and particular pain of a severe and potentially terminal illness, Jimmy Anderson and his mother evolved a definition of "normalcy" personal to the situation, in spite of, perhaps in defiance of, what was taking place.

Remarkably, despite his worn-down condition, Jimmy did not lose his peppery personality or his sense of humor. He had a beautiful full smile, a spray of freckles across his nose, and a repertoire of antics. Once, at church, to the smiling chagrin of his family, he nonchalantly told the usher passing the collection tray, "I gave at the office."

He also liked to play jokes. He would occasionally telephone his grandmother, Anne's mother, for example, of whom he was especially fond, and try to drop his boyish voice down to the pitch of a grown man's. Pretending to be his uncle, he would say in a gravelly tenor, "Hello Nanna, this is your son, Frank." His grandmother would easily go along, asking him how things were at the office. Then Jimmy would laugh.

When he was feeling strong, he would sometimes help his mother prepare supper, cutting up vegetables or stirring a cake or a batch of brownies. When there was time, the two would cap an afternoon with a board game like Chutes and Ladders or a hand of cards. Life was for the most part circumscribed by what Jimmy could do at home. The entire house became his sickroom, and his mother became, of necessity, his best and closest friend. It was a kind of repetition of the bonding that takes place between mother and child at birth, except instead of celebrating the full promise of life, the bond is based on keeping life from being snatched away.

In Anne Anderson's words, "Sometimes I wanted to help him so much, I did not know where he ended and I began. We were together all the time. He became an extension of me."

And so she remembers the day of the mayor's meeting particularly well because it was one of those rare days when Jimmy was not at home. The house was totally silent, save for Anne's movements around the kitchen and laundry and bath, until the phone rang and a teacher from Jimmy's school told her Jimmy had forgotten his lunch. She drove across Woburn to the special school he was attending—he suffered a slight learning and fine motor control disability as a result of his early radiation treatments—thinking it was too bad he could not have had at least one uninterruptedly ordinary day. On the way back home she drove past city hall and thought about the meeting with the mayor that was probably going on at that moment. The image triggered her frustrations and she says, "All of a sudden I felt this rush of rage about what was happening to Jimmy and that nothing was being done to find out what might have caused it." She drove home, ran into her bedroom, and changed into clothes suitable for a mayoral meeting.

She reached city hall with the conference still in full swing. She identified herself simply as a member of FACE and was shown into the spacious office dominated by a large, dark wooden desk. The mayor was in the middle of a sentence when she entered and did not stop. Her friends, including Bruce Young, nodded at her but did not introduce her. She sat in a chair behind the others, not sure what she would say now that she had come. The mayor stopped talking and said to no one in particular, "and who is this?" Anne heard herself say her name quietly, that she lived in East Woburn, and without mentioning leukemia, or Jimmy, she added, "I think you should know there are people in my neighborhood who are very upset." As the meeting was breaking up the mayor spoke to Bruce Young in the hall and said forcefully, "You see. This is what I mean—this hysteria. This is what I am afraid of."

The mayor had been expressing concern to Young that the public attention FACE was bringing to the toxic waste problem might cause panic in the community, in particular, panic in the real estate market. The mayor did not say a direct word to Anne or offer a regret about the illness of her son. "I felt like the invisible woman," she remembers. The meeting adjourned, and FACE continued its efforts.

Between January and early June 1980 no official investigations of the leukemia cluster were made.

By then, however, toxic waste was a major national issue, and Senator Kennedy's office had become deeply involved in drafting the Comprehensive Environmental Response Compensation and Liability Act, known as Superfund, which was aimed at providing funds for cleanup of the major sites. Kennedy chaired the Subcommittee on Health and Scientific Research of the Senate Committees on Labor, Human Resources, and the Judiciary. He asked Bruce Young, Anne Anderson, and Judy Broderick of Reading, Massachusetts, an adjacent town where the Woburn smell reached, to testify at hearings on health effects of hazardous waste disposal practices.

It was a good opportunity to focus congressional attention on the concrete individual problems of health and toxic waste, but Anne Anderson was still somewhat timid about public speaking. At the hearings on June 6, Bruce Young did most of the talking. He laid out the facts he and Anne had gathered and provided copies of the map he and Anne had made. He told the packed hearing room, hot from an early summer, "For seven years we were told that the burden of proof was upon us as independent citizens to gather the statistics. . . . All our work was done independent of the Commonwealth of Massachusetts. They offered no support, were in fact one of our adversaries in this battle to prove that we had a problem. And the intention going in was just to find the facts: was there indeed a cluster of leukemia in East Woburn, or was there not? It was incumbent upon us to do that work."

Young continued, explaining the materials he had brought along, "What you should be aware of in the coding of that map, those figures in black represent deaths; those colored in green are children that are still living. And the Commonwealth of Massachusetts only goes on mortality, so because those children have not died yet, they are not important in their statistical analysis." He meant, of course, there was not as yet any tumor registry in Massachusetts and consequently no way to stay current on the incidence of any type of cancer, let alone childhood leukemia.

The Senate subcommittee also heard Dr. David Rall, then director of the National Institute of Environmental Health Sciences, on what it takes to respond to the questions about environment and health that Bruce Young had outlined. "The medical community moves slowly. Let me remind you all of the problem with cigarette smoking. There was a study by Doll and Hill in 1952, looking at 35,000 people, that showed cancer linked to cigarette smoke. It was not until 1976 that the surgeon general came out with his report. Things just move slowly when you go through the sort of channel that demands a kind of ultimate proof."

James McCarthy, of Jackson Township, New Jersey, thirty-three years old, also testified. He described the health picture in the rural neighborhood called Legler about a mile downstream from a toxic waste landfill that had been found to be leaking chemicals, including TCE, into a 4–square mile area and consequently contaminating the groundwater that fed wells serving eight houses, including McCarthy's. His community at the time was purchasing all of its drinking water privately, and because the town of Jackson had thus far not connected his area to the municipal system, contaminated groundwater continued to be the neighborhood's only source of bath water.

The homes in Legler were set in a row, and eight people from six homes had serious kidney problems, including two who had had to have kidneys removed—McCarthy was one—and two persons who were on dialysis. Kidney problems are of particular interest in cases of toxic exposure because it is the kidney that must work arduously to either purify or excrete from the body substances not meant to be inside it. McCarthy added to his list seven miscarriages, a mysterious sudden infant death, and recurrent vaginal infections among women and eye problems among all. And then McCarthy, thirty-three years old, reared on the tough streets of Brooklyn, New York, wept openly when he told the committee of the death of his nine-month-old daughter from a rare kidney cancer.

In all, ten witnesses from towns in Massachusetts, New Jersey, New York, and Tennessee spoke of mysterious illnesses in neighborhoods within the orbit of a major toxic waste site. And all testified that they had, so far, been given no satisfactory explanations for the problems or assurances that answers were being sought. In every case the burden of establishing that a problem existed had fallen on the citizens in question.

The hearing culminated with all parties being clear that no one agency in government had the resources or authority to get to the bottom of clusters of adverse health effects, let alone uncover them in the first place, and that between the EPA, the CDC, the NIH, and the HEW, responsibility had fallen. None of the witnesses, however, had taken their private investigations as far as Bruce Young and Anne Anderson had. The hearings, including Mr. McCarthy's tears, made the evening television news, the *New York Times*, and the *Washington Post*.

About two weeks later, during the week of May 23, the CDC and the National Institute of Occupational Safety and Health (NIOSH) sent Dr. John Cutler, a staff epidemiologist, to Woburn to supervise a team of interviewers affiliated with the Massachusetts Department of Public Health. The goal was to verify that a true cluster of leukemia existed, as well as to determine overall cancer incidence in Woburn.

NIOSH had gotten involved in Woburn because it had learned through a member of the Woburn community that three persons at least—all former workers in a pet food plant in Woburn—were suffering from kidney cancer, an unusually high number for a plant work force of less than a thousand.

The investigating team began to carry out the standard epidemiological case-control study in which a group thought to have a factor in common is compared with a "control" group similar in every way to the case group. Interviewers talked with one or both parents of the twelve children diagnosed with leukemia who appeared on the map Bruce Young and Anne Anderson had devised. By then, eight of the children had died. Each leukemia case had two matched "controls"—a child who lived near the leukemic child and one who lived much further away. For this study a "case" was defined as a confirmed victim of kidney cancer, liver cancer, urinary tract or bladder cancer, or leukemia in a child under nineteen years of age.

The questionnaire was lengthy and asked age, ethnic background, diagnosis, onset of symptoms, past medical history, pregnancy history of mother, father's military history, family background, smoking history, residential history, occupational history, and several questions about environmental exposures including gardening habits, contact with farm animals, diet, activities near dump sites, or open bodies of water in Woburn, and exposure to specific chemicals including hair spray and hair dye.

Anne Anderson and her family answered the questions carefully when the CDC investigative team came to her home, but at no time was she asked any questions outside of those which appeared on the questionnaire. She says her opinion about cause, or that of any parent of a leukemic child, were not solicited. In fact, Anne Anderson was the last parent to be questioned; she says she was told her family had almost been inadvertently overlooked.

The questionnaire data was collected, but it could not be compared to any standard overall list of leukemia cases because incidence records were not kept at the time by the state or anyone else. The CDC internal memo summarizing its work in Woburn refers to the fact that Dr. John Truman and Reverend Young—Anne Anderson's name does not appear—supplied the initial information on leukemia incidence. CDC investigators also consulted with two referral hospitals, hospitals to which cancer cases were generally referred, for further data.

And it cited another alert individual. Because a local pathologist had notified the Massachusetts Department of Public Health that he felt he had seen and heard about an increased number of bladder tumor tissue specimens, the CDC was able to identify six more kidney cancer cases and twenty-nine more cases of bladder cancer.

The CDC investigation lasted through the summer, and in the meantime, Jimmy Anderson's condition badly deteriorated. He had been removed from chemotherapy late in the spring, and the hope was that the leukemia would stay in remission. But he grew especially weak and run down and increasingly unable to maintain even his own scaled-down program of activities. Every now and then he would call his problem "leukenia" and say he wished he did not have it.

In fact at this point he did not. The leukemia cells remained in check, but his mother sensed life was slipping away from him nevertheless. That summer he was diagnosed with aplastic anemia, a disease of the bone marrow that prevents the production of red blood cells needed to carry oxygen and platelets needed for clotting. The powerful drugs aimed at the leukemia cells can also shut down the basic cell-producing mechanism—the bone marrow—altogether, since treatment can obliterate the stem cells from which the normal blood components grow. Radiation can have the same effect. Once the last seed cells die, aplastic anemia results. Anemia is a risk of leukemia treatment.

But as bad as aplastic anemia can be, that diagnosis was a relief to the Andersons compared to the news they might have had that the dreaded leukemia cells had reappeared. The Andersons again went to Epping for the summer. Even though it was a logistic nightmare for Anne, coordinating summer camp for her son Chuck and hospital visits for Jimmy, she felt that on balance Jimmy always had a better time when he was in Epping.

But this summer brought an extra pressure, for Charles Anderson had decided to separate from his wife. He had been offered a position with his firm in their Toronto office, and he wanted his family to move with him. But Anne had been reluctant to do so, mostly because she felt strongly that Jimmy should remain in John Truman's care. He knew Jimmy's case well, and she felt his personal sensitivity and warmth toward Jimmy were crucial to the boy's chances for recovery.

But it was more than a matter of location and doctors. The long years of stress on the family had strained the Anderson marriage passed a point where it could be redeemed. Anne felt she had been presented with an untenable choice between her marriage and her son. Charles felt that Anne was unfairly characterizing the situation, for he insisted Jimmy could receive excellent treatment in Toronto as well. They could not communicate, and they could not compromise. Charles Anderson left.

Pressure began to build on another front, for the media attention on Woburn did not abate. A major story in the *Boston Globe* called Woburn a "tangle of dumps and disease," and a roving columnist in the *Woburn Daily Times* wrote a story called "Can Public Relations Save the Day." It began: "Wanted: Public relations expert to change image of medium-size city in midst of toxic waste crisis."

Since the testimony in Washington before the Ken-

edy subcommittee, Anne Anderson and Bruce Young
were besieged with calls from newspapers and television
networks. Reporters began to prowl East Woburn trying
to locate the Anderson house.

Anne, ambivalent over what to tell Jimmy about their
sudden prominence, told him that his case was special
because people might be able to learn from it. Once or
twice she consented to his being interviewed directly.
But she never again did because one day a news crew,
when they happened to see Jimmy struggle weakly to
get out of a taxi, asked him to do it again for television.
Later that week, even though he knew that what had
happened to him had started something important in
Woburn, he wrote his mother a note that said, "Mom,
I hat cameras."

Things got worse into the fall and holiday season.
Treatments with hormones had not reversed the anemia, and Jimmy was in constant danger of hemorrhage,
for his blood was simply not clotting properly. He would
bleed spontaneously from his nose, his gums, his ears.
Regularly he would have to be transfused with platelets
and blood to keep the internal bleeding under control.
During this period, Anne Anderson never knew on beginning a day whether it would end without a trip to
the hospital. Carol Gray often came to the Andersons on
a moment's notice if Jimmy began to bleed either to
help Anne get him to the hospital or to help keep tabs
on the welfare of Chuck and Christine, who though free
of leukemia, nevertheless shared its impact through its
effect on Jimmy.

Christine Anderson was nine years old when Jimmy
was diagnosed, but she has no memories of family life

before the diagnosis. "It just doesn't seem that there was much before that," she says.

But despite the leukemia, Christine found ways to play with Jimmy, sometimes at his expense she admits with an embarrassed smile. Such as the occasion when she and a girlfriend would dress him up in outlandish costumes—one day a shepherd, one day a doll—and he would be a willing participant, glad for the company and the break from routine. And as he grew older, now and then Jimmy would bring up the subject of death and ask his sister what she thought it might be like.

As Jimmy grew older, Christine was increasingly relied upon at home to do the shopping or to prepare supper if her mother had to be at the hospital. Once when Jimmy was hospitalized, he asked for a bowl of spaghetti topped with his mother's tomato sauce. Anne couldn't leave the hospital, and so Chris tried to make the sauce, cooking three batches until she felt she had it tasting right. Still, she confesses to being torn between loyalty to brother and her own urge to be free to grow up.

She does, however, have very real and fond memories of times when Jimmy was well enough to go out, and he would be nearly ecstatic at the chance to go with her to the grocery store for a quart of milk. "About the best he ever felt," she said, "was once when my boyfriend, Kevin, and I took him shopping in Kevin's car. He sat on Kevin's lap and Kevin let him pretend to be driving. It made Jimmy so happy. It almost made me think he was going to be all right."

Charles Anderson, Jr., or Chuckie, was only two years older than Jimmy, and the two boys shared a room. The mention of his brother's name can bring quiet to Chuck's eyes. "I can remember Jimmy almost always lying on the couch in the living room or in bed," he said, glancing around the room as he described it. "Jimmy's bed was right here, and lots of times he would be awake when I would come in, and he would throw things at me and me at him. We tried to be regular brothers." Like Christine, Chuck was a raring-to-go adolescent as the limitations of Jimmy's illness unfolded. Though Chuck did spend time keeping Jimmy company, he also remembers many a day when he would look back at the window in time to see Jimmy looking out, waving. "Once," Chuck recalls, "my mother took us shopping and bought us each a model plane. I came home and put mine in my room and got ready to go play hockey. Jimmy was really tired after shopping and got into his bed. He started looking at the model, and I realized he was too weak to put it together. I told my friends to go on without me, and I came back into the room and helped Jim. It made his day, that we could make those models together. It was about the best thing I could ever do for my brother."

In December 1980, Jimmy was admitted to Massachusetts General. He was exceedingly thin, too sick to eat normally, having had the yen for favorite foods such as spaghetti, Big Macs, and roast chicken with stuffing, but never any stamina to eat them. At one point he had to have a blood transfusion every three or four days, and Dr. Truman or the nurses characterized his urine tests to his mother in terms of color—"like rosé wine, like tea," reflecting the amount of internal blood. Soon Jimmy's veins were too collapsed to support the transfusing needles. A plastic line was inserted through Jimmy's chest so blood, blood products, and medicine could be administered to him that way. He also had to endure a similar tube to his stomach, which was used to feed him, the standard intravenous system no longer being usable because of his weakened veins. The tubes were capped when Jimmy was not connected to a piece of equipment.

Dr. Truman allowed Jimmy to come home for twenty-four hours at Christmas, and the family tried to make the best of the circumstances. By this time Jimmy weighed much less than 50 pounds, but still he kept up his fight for life. When he left home to return to the hospital for the last time, he just put his hand in his mother's and said nothing, made no complaint, as if to steel himself and the others for what lay ahead.

Anne Anderson moved into the hospital, sleeping in Jimmy's room. "Jimmy looked like a puppet," she says, "he was hooked up to so many lines." Visitors were constant, nevertheless.

As Jimmy Anderson's health had been deteriorating, epidemiological work on the cluster had continued. On January 23, 1981, the Massachusetts Department of Public Health released the report it had completed with the assistance of the CDC. It concluded that there were indeed twelve cases of childhood leukemia in East Woburn, where 5.3 would have been expected or normal for the period of time and size of the population involved. Of the twelve cases, nine were boys, where 3.1 cases among males would be expected. The report confirmed that nine of the twelve cases were of the acute lymphocytic type, with the others chronic monocytic, acute monocytic, and acute myelocytic, respectively. Eight of the twelve children had lived in Woburn all their lives. Two had lived there since the age of one. The cases were concentrated in East Woburn, and six lived within or on the border of one census tract, which is to say within a half-mile radius. They were literally a dozen or so houses apart. The odds of six cases living so close together by chance alone were roughly 100 to 1.

Kidney cancer was also confirmed to be elevated in Woburn and tended to concentrate in the area around Horn Pond, another body of water in Woburn.

The discussion of the findings was inconclusive. The report said, "The case-control study failed to identify any factor that significantly distinguished the cases from the controls. This is not altogether surprising for, with few exceptions, investigations of leukemia clusters have failed to demonstrate significant associations or even promising leads as to possible environmental causes." The report continued that "possibly of [more] relevance to the leukemia concentration is the contamination of wells G and H. . . . As far as we have been able to determine, environmental data do not exist prior to 1979 that would give us any indication of what, if any, contaminants existed in wells G and H in the past . . . the lack of environmental data for earlier periods is a major obstacle in trying to establish a link between environmental variables and the health effects identified in Woburn."

The report also said "Findings that childhood leukemia became elevated in the eastern part of Woburn only after wells G and H came on line would support the hypothesis that the elevated leukemia incidence was related to drinking water contamination. . . . Well G was on line during the probable critical exposure period for the leukemia cases some time prior to diagnosis, which for most of these children was the mid to late 1960s. . . . It is important to stress that the contaminants [TCE et al.] found in wells G and H are not known to cause leukemia. Yet the fact that organic contaminants were found at all in the water supply must also be emphasized."

The report added that "the hypothesis suggesting that the increase in leukemia incidence was associated with environmental hazards in Woburn, and specifically with the contamination of drinking water supplies, is neither supported nor refuted by the study findings."

These words came nearly a decade after Jimmy Anderson's diagnosis and Anne Anderson's first suspicion about the leukemia cluster. And with news of the study results, networks reran any taped interviews of Jimmy they could locate. Anne Anderson watched with sad recognition the sight of her son on television. For five days prior to the release of the report, on January 18, 1981, at Massachusetts General Hospital, Jimmy Anderson had quietly died.

10

"The Available Technology Was Unable to Determine..."

DEATH CAN SEEM a straightforward matter until it envelops a child, for the death of a child is a shocking event. It flouts the natural expectation that a child is born to outlive his parents, that new generations replace the old. Instead, especially if the child has died of a long illness, parents are left with memories of the sad innocent struggle their child tried to mount against the inherently more powerful force of death. There can be nothing straightforward about something so patently unfair.

The direct cause of Jimmy Anderson's death was massive pulmonary hemorrhage, a heavy bleeding in his lungs that could not be stopped and that ultimately suffocated him. The aplastic anemia had been the underlying cause of the bleeding, and it in turn had been brought on by the long years of chemotherapy.

Ultimately, Jimmy had simply wasted away. Born weighing 10½ pounds, and 22½ inches long, he never weighed more than 52 pounds in his life and was less than 50 inches tall when he died. As Jimmy's doctor, John Truman, pointed out, "The very saddest thing about Jimmy's case is that he died not from the disease

174

but from the treatment." Echoing the irony of the cluster itself, he adds, "It's rare, but it can happen."

Whether Jimmy's condition was worsened by the fact that he had been unknowingly exposed to contaminated water at home for most of the years he was being treated can never be known.

The deaths of children are what knit some of the Woburn community together. When the Anderson family held a memorial service for Jimmy several days after his death, the crowd was overflowing from the church. Joan and Pat Zona attended, just as Anne Anderson had attended the funeral of their son, Michael, who died of leukemia in 1974. By late January 1981, nine of the twelve children in the original cluster, including Jimmy, had died.

The collective sense of loss attending these events is practically inexpressible. Healing takes an especially long period of time and may never be fully achieved, because losing a child is a tragedy and experience for which the human psyche is totally unprepared.

If such an event shatters one's balance, in Woburn where parents suspected a controllable force was implicated in the deaths, such an event also shakes one's belief in the effectiveness of institutions in which one is predisposed to have faith. In the case of Woburn, science failed to convince the parents who were looking for an explanation that they were wrong. A layperson's approach to epidemiological science evolved, perhaps even as an internalized reaction to grief, but based on intelligent reasonable thinking nevertheless. Rage and sadness over the death of their children is what moved Woburn parents, particularly Anne Anderson, to act.

Professional institutions do not generally respond to an amateur's thinking, regardless of motive. As Nicholas Paleologos, the young Massachusetts state representative put it, "it was like a virtuoso being approached by someone who has just found classical music and all of a sudden wants to talk Bach. At the time the Woburn events were unfolding, the public health and scientific establishment in Boston was not ready for people in Woburn traipsing around, finding things, reading articles, learning, asking questions about viruses and carcinogens."

It was not, however, as though the Woburn cluster was alone at the time. Woburn broke into the news right in the middle of several similar investigations at other places around the country. For example, in 1978, before it was known that toxic wastes were present in Woburn and before the existence of the cluster had been established, Rutherford, New Jersey, had become the target of a cluster investigation eerily suggestive of the Woburn situation.

The town itself is physically similar. It is located 6 miles west of New York City in Bergen County near the swampy areas called the Meadowlands. There is a little industry in Rutherford itself, but the town lies in the industrial corridor of New Jersey, which is a center of petrochemical and other chemical production. Fumes, smoke, and waste dumps have been an undeniable element of Rutherford's general environment for decades, according to residents, although there is no specific locus, like wells G and H or the Industri-Plex site.

Most of Rutherford's approximately 21,000 people live in sturdy, large but not imposing one-family homes, which were built when the cost of heating such houses never entered the mind. The town's Main Street is long and busy, similar to Woburn's in that one senses that malls and shopping centers are slowly but surely sucking commerce away from what was once a vital heart. Nevertheless, touches of small town ways remain. On Valentine's Day, for example, a local card shop sells handwritten copies of "How do I love thee." The public library serves also as an exchange depot for grocery coupons; a box of them sits on a table near the library entrance with a small sign saying "take a few and leave a few." Rutherford is clean, and there are plenty of trees. It is quiet, middle-class, and pleasant.

In March of 1978 a mother, Vivian Cleffi, whose son has subsequently died of leukemia, wrote the Rutherford Board of Education calling its attention to the fact that there seemed to be several cases of leukemia among children who attended the Pierrepont Elementary School, the town's largest public school, which served about 540 students in grades kindergarten through six. The Board referred the letter to Henry McCafferty, who heads the town's health department, who then called state health officials, who in turn alerted the Centers for Disease Control in Atlanta.

As it would in Woburn, the research first sought to verify the parent's instinct and to officially establish the number of cases involved. Eventually thirteen leukemia cases were confirmed, six in the age group nineteen and under and seven over age nineteen. According to the report published by the CDC and New Jersey Department of Health officials, "the location of the homes of the leukemia cases suggests a cluster among the leukemia cases less than nineteen years of age but not among the older cases. All school-age children with leukemia lived in the school district." Analysis of the data revealed a "significantly increased incidence of childhood leukemia in the Pierrepont School District" (although not all the sick children were attending the school at the time their illness appeared). Nine cases of Hodgkin's disease were also confirmed, an incidence found to be "significantly higher" than what would be expected for the twenty to thirty-nine age group, but the geographical locations of the Hodgkin's cases did not suggest clustering. Once the "significance" of the incidence had been established, bearing out the parent's original suspicion, investigators set out to find a cause, although McCafferty himself told the newspapers he doubted a cause would be found. Dr. Ronald Altman, an epidemiologist with the state of New Jersey who was called in on the case, addressed a public meeting of 700 residents with the same realistic, if discouraging, message.

The investigators distributed a questionnaire to all families with a leukemia or Hodgkin's disease case, as well as to a randomly selected control group. The questionnaire solicited the standard demographic information, and gauged environmental factors such as the respondee's exposure to microwave ovens, house extermination, tree spraying, paint stripping, benzene, shampoo, household insecticides and pets, including gerbils. In an unusual move urged by the community the New Jersey Department of Environmental Protection also took air samples at the Pierrepont School. Brick scrapings from the school were also tested for low-level radiation and other contaminants, as was the town water supply. But from all the questions and the testing nothing was found that might explain the cluster.

The epidemiologic investigation concluded, in a paper published in April 1980, with the familiar language, "many apparent clusters will occur by chance alone. The available technology was unable to determine if the excess disease incidence represented a chance event or a case unique to Rutherford." Benzene, a known leukemogen, was found to be the most prevalent air pollutant found in Rutherford, but in amounts that could not be considered "abnormal" according to the report.

The environmental investigators concluded, in an accompanying paper, "several carcinogenic substances were found in low concentrations in the Rutherford environment. However, given the present state of knowledge about the etiology of Hodgkin's disease and leukemia, and the effects of low-level exposure to carcinogens, it is impossible to link the presence of these substances to the clusters." The words might have been written about Woburn, and they had been written in conjunction with the CDC, but neither Bruce Young nor Anne Anderson received information about these other similar situations from the CDC representatives who talked with them or from their own Massachusetts Department of Public Health.

Toxic waste was not the only potential culprit in these other potential clusters. Take the case of Erwin, Tennessee, for example. Erwin, in Unicoi County, was home to a nuclear fuel processing plant which admitted that prior to 1977 it discharged radioactive wastes into a local creek. The creek then flowed to the Nolichucky

River. Residents of Unicoi were exposed to airborne radioactive wastes, while residents downstream from the plant in Washington County drew their drinking water from the river. To boot, the Erwin plant was chronically missing the highly toxic radioactive material plutonium. This radioactive fuel, which is in theory parsimoniously doled out to plants, could not be accounted for in the regular accounting procedures designed to keep track of the substances. Plant officials said they could not explain where the missing material went and said it was probably "lost in the pipes." (In fact, the plant was so often missing nuclear material that the legal maximum level such plants could report as "unaccounted for" was raised by the Nuclear Regulatory Commission in January 1980—just so Erwin, which produces nuclear submarine fuel, could remain in operation.)

In any case, in April 1978, before the Woburn news had broken, but after the Rutherford cluster had been identified, an article in the *Atlanta Constitution* reported that there had been a twofold increase in cancer deaths in Unicoi County. However, in August 1979 when the CDC reported on its findings, it said that when the effect of aging in the population was taken into statistical account, no "statistically significant" increase in cancer incidence was noted, although in more or less the same breath the CDC did note that leukemia and respiratory deaths were "in excess of expected." The CDC concluded "while epidemiologists can effectively evaluate large clusters, large changes in rate, or major exposure problems, they can do little to assess a small increase in the incidence of a disease or a small potential risk to a population."

Also in 1978 and 1979, CDC researchers were putting the finishing touches on a paper based on an investigation made in rural Mississippi, Arkansas, and Tennessee, where thirteen adolescents had been diagnosed with a rare colorectal adenocarcinoma, cancer of the lower bowels, between September 1974 and November 1976. None of the children had a family history of this type of cancer, not even a history of colitis. Ten of the children lived in agricultural areas of the Mississippi Delta where pesticide use was high, and seven of the children had a documentable history of exposure to pesticides by virtue of the intensive farming under way just near where they lived. Yet, according to the CDC report, published in the journal *Cancer*, "Serum levels of pesticide residues in this small number of cases, however, do not give any support to the hypothesis that exposure to pesticides may have caused this apparent regional increase in cases of colorectal adenocarcinoma, although three individual families had high levels."

Though the Rutherford, Unicoi, and rural Mississippi cases had all been handled through the same office of the CDC, the parallel nature of the situations was never brought to the attention of the families in the leukemia cluster while the CDC was compiling its report on Woburn. It was only as Bruce Young and Anne Anderson and other For A Clean Environment (FACE) members took it upon themselves to learn more about what a "cluster" actually was, that they became aware of the constant and chronic frustration attendant to unraveling them.

But as they tried to understand a cluster as a theoretical, intellectual phenomenon, they were again confronted with its at-hand concrete meaning. In the late winter of 1981, a month or so after Jimmy Anderson's death, Patrick Toomey's condition worsened. He had been born in June 1969 and diagnosed on August 15, 1979, with leukemia. He lived on Wood Street, about a three-minute drive from the Andersons. He had been responding to treatment, and in December 1980, as Jimmy Anderson was dying, Patrick seemed healthy again, sporting a full head of deep brown hair and a bright flash of a smile. But by March of 1981, Patrick was bedridden, a rail of a child intuitively aware he was facing death, trying to say things he thought would make his parents feel better.

The Toomeys set up Patrick's bed in their living room so it would be easier for him to feel a part of the household, although he could not walk freely around the house anymore. This was around the time that preliminary inspections of the Industri-Plex site were being made with an eye toward figuring out what to do about it, and when Senator Edward Kennedy visited the site late in March, he also took the opportunity to visit the Toomey family. Kennedy shook the press and town officials and walked up the slightly graded front yard without an entourage. Mrs. Toomey offered him a cup of tea and a plate of cookies, which he accepted, and he spent about an hour talking alone with Patrick. He was the only public official to actually meet with any of the children in the cluster, and the visit left him visibly shaken and tearful.

On March 25, the Toomeys, devout Roman Catholics, accepted their priest's offer to say a mass at Patrick's bedside. Patrick had loved being an altar boy, and some of the boys with whom he served also attended this mass. Later that night, a few months before his twelfth birthday, Patrick Toomey died.

Anne Anderson and many others attended the funeral service—Patrick's death on the heels of Jimmy's. For Anne Anderson, relieved of the daily pressure of caring for a dying child, Patrick's death only amplified the sequence and the implications of her long-held suspicions. Deeply frustrated and emotionally drained, Anne Anderson half-withdrew from life, remaining composed in public, but still, for example, able to say only "the back room," "the spare room," "the other room," but never yet "Jimmy's room." She did not "get away" as friends recommended, but instead tried to keep life going for her two remaining children.

However, publicity and politics were beginning to latch on to the findings she and Bruce Young had put forward. The Woburn events began to assume a life of their own.

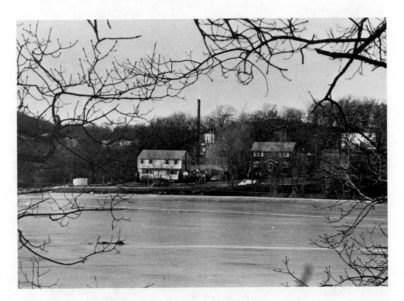

East Woburn neighborhood with Walker Pond and tannery smoke-stack.

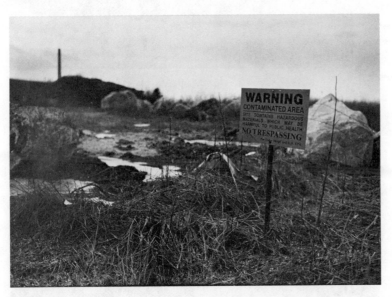

Industri-Plex toxic waste dump in northeast Woburn.

(Photographs on pp. 185, 186, and 188 to 194 by Carrie Boretz.)

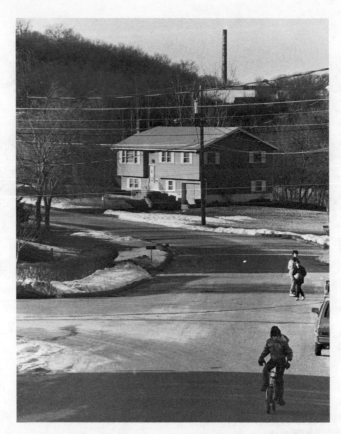

A street in East Woburn.

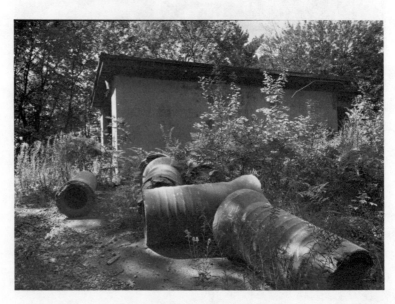

Abandoned station of well G.

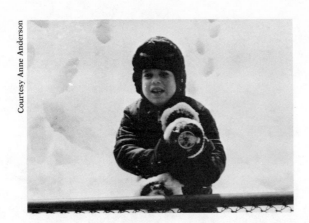

Jimmy Anderson, three and a half years old, shortly after diagnosis.

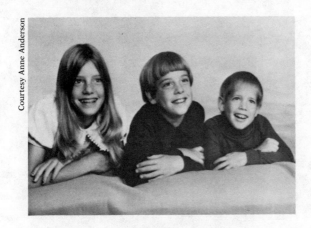

Christine, Charles, Jr., and Jimmy Anderson (Jimmy, age four).

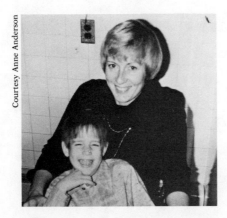

Anne Anderson with son Jimmy (Jimmy, age nine).

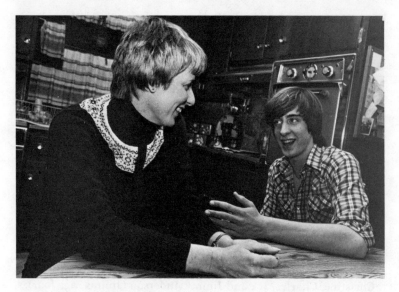

Anne Anderson with son Chuck (1984).

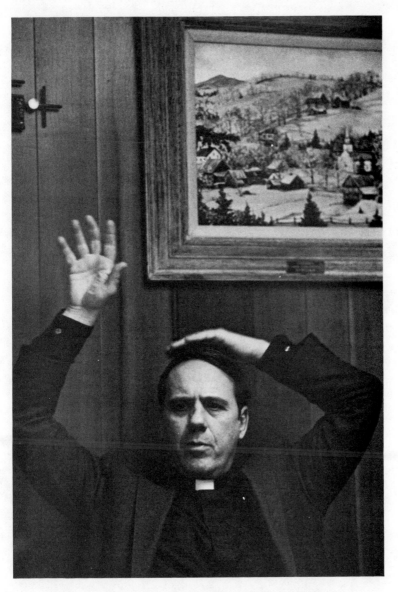

Rev. Bruce C. Young in his office at Trinity Church.

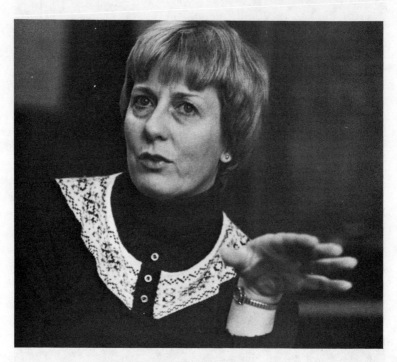

Anne Anderson, 1984.

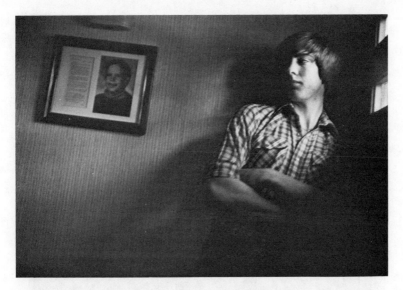

Chuck Anderson with photo of Jimmy.

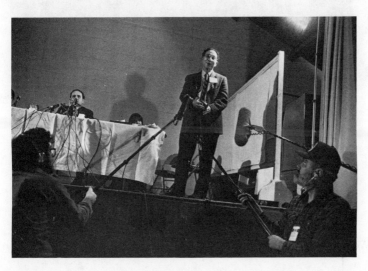

Dr. Marvin Zelen, February 1984, at Trinity Church announcing results of Harvard biostatistics department study on wells G and H and
leukemia.

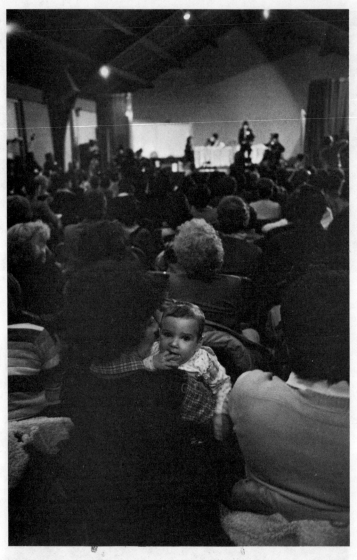

Woburn Community at meeting on February 8, 1984. Zellen talking.

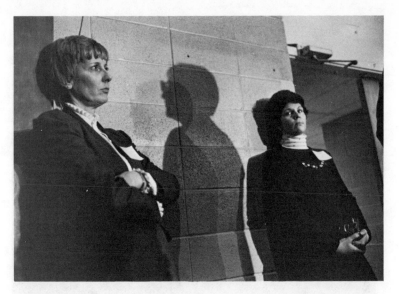

Anne Anderson and Donna Robbins listening to Harvard results.

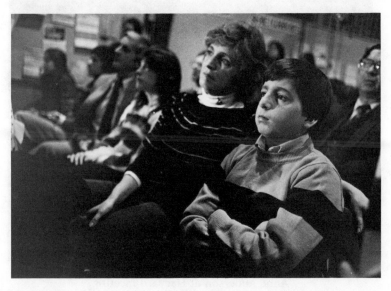

Kevin Kane, Jr., and family (mother Patricia and father and sister in background) at meeting on results of Harvard study.

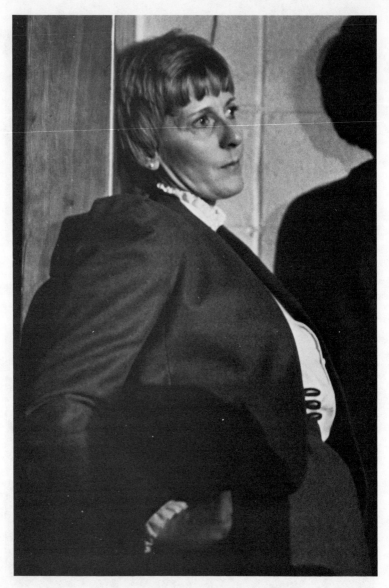

Anne Anderson at Harvard meeting.

11

The New Detectives

IN THE SPRING of 1981 Anne Anderson and Bruce Young were invited by Dr. Larry Brown of the Community Health Improvement Program of the Harvard University School of Public Health to describe the Woburn events at a seminar for faculty and students. Located in a gray, polished slate building in the Brookline section of Boston, the school is one of the most prestigious academic institutions of its kind in the world.

It was only a few months after Jimmy Anderson's death, and Anne Anderson did not feel up to the trip to Brookline or to speaking about his illness yet another time. But Bruce Young convinced her that this would be an audience from which they might learn and which, he felt, ought to hear about Woburn in detail from those who knew the story best.

Students and faculty from the school attended the seminar, and Anderson and Young carefully outlined the chronology of events, describing their own amateur detective work over the previous several years. They vented some of their frustration at how difficult it was to develop "proof" there really was a cluster and "proof" of what might have caused it, and they described in personal terms their experiences with attempting to en-

195

gage the continuing interest of public health authorities. Bruce Young remembers feeling at the time, "I just couldn't believe it was going to end with the MDPH and CDC study, that it could just stop there. I didn't know why there weren't scientists crawling all over the town trying to get to the bottom of what happened. I thought we could be a proverbial living laboratory for finding out about causes of leukemia."

Dr. Marvin Zelen, chairman of the school's biostatistics department, was part of the seminar audience. Formerly associated with the National Cancer Institute, he is a leading biostatistician, a practitioner of the science of using statistics to track and determine trends in health and medical treatment. No stranger to the demography of cancer, Zelen's most recent biostatistical focus had been on evaluating the efficacy of specific kinds of cancer treatments. By studying which patients with which types of cancer were receiving which types of chemotherapy and for how long and whether they survived, Zelen had become an expert at using statistics to determine whether the treatments were truly effective or whether survival rates were quirks and unrelated to a particular drug at all.

Zelen listened carefully to the Woburn talk. His is the understated realm of probability and shades of likelihood, but he remembers being "very moved" by the presentation of the lists of leukemia cases and the history of tracking them down. He had heard, of course, about the extent of the toxic waste in Woburn and about the closing of the wells, but he had not been aware before of the potential relationship between the environmental situation in Woburn and the leukemia cases. The predicament tapped his professional curiosity. "To some extent I was excited," he says, objectively measuring his words, "by a fascinating intellectual problem. On the one hand, the kids, the leukemia, the wells. On the other, the legitimate possibility that nothing more than chance was involved."

The seminar ended. Spring grew warmer. Robbie Robbins, diagnosed with leukemia in 1976, was now nine years old and, though weak and encumbered by his leg brace, was able to play a modified version of baseball the neighborhood kids called teeball. One day in June he took his position at bat and connected firmly with the ball. His mother sat on the sidelines with a crowd of parents, and the players in the field slowed down in order to give Robbie, whom they knew at minimum was "sick," a chance to make it around the bases. He crossed home plate a home-run hitter.

He ran to his mother and practically collapsed at her feet, completely out of breath. She did not know then that his red blood count had been dropping precipitously because the leukemia cells were overwhelming his healthy red cells again and that Robbie had been growing increasingly anemic. She took Robbie right into the hospital, where he received an emergency transfusion. He remained in a precarious situation all summer and was in and out of the hospital. He grew increasingly weak and spent a good deal of the time when he was out of the hospital dependent on a wheelchair.

On August 15, 1981, however, Robbie Robbins died.

Donna Robbins, like the Toomeys and some of the other parents of leukemic children, had remained somewhat skeptical of a link between the water and the leu-

kemias. But as news of the possibility of toxic contamination had become public through 1979 and 1980, their
skepticism had waned. With Jimmy's death, then Patrick's, and now Robbie's, opinions had begun to seal
among the Woburn parents.

By midsummer, Marvin Zelen and his associate, Dr.
Steven Lagakos, another biostatistician, who seems as
comfortable with numbers as it is possible for a human
being to be, had reviewed what was known scientifically
thus far about the Woburn events. Lagakos too had been
drawn to the statistical challenge Woburn represented,
and the possibility that biostatistics could add to the
body of knowledge.

It was an intriguing situation, for no cluster investigation had ever been able to get beyond merely confirming "statistical significance," that is, confirming
that the bump in the line of normalcy a cluster represented was indeed abnormal. That had already been
done in Woburn, but no one was further along toward understanding whether this statistically significant cluster had a cause unrelated to chance.

In fact, a follow-up report by the MDPH issued in
November of 1981 seemed only to contradict the statistical work the department had published the previous
January. The second report said, "One of the purposes
of this study was to test further whether there was an
association between the use of water from wells G and
H and the occurrence of leukemia. These additional data
seem to weaken this association. The number of childhood leukemia deaths began to rise in the 1959–1963
period, before the wells were drilled, and continued to
rise in the period in which the wells were drilled. Given

an average latent period of two to five years, childhood leukemia associated with wells G and H should not have started to increase until 1969–73, when in fact, the rate was lower than expected. The very small number of childhood leukemia deaths, 14 over 30 years, precludes any strong statistical conclusion."

Despite the report's tentative tone, however, it had been preceded by a widely disseminated press release that was much firmer in its choice of words: "Contamination of two wells that served eastern Woburn during the 1960's and 1970's probably did not cause that area's high rate of childhood leukemia, according to a new M.D.P.H. study."

Thus despite what had been billed as a follow-up study, the community of Woburn was still largely in the dark about what had caused the leukemia cluster.

Any cluster investigations are subject to the inherent limitations of the statistical research process itself. One major drawback is the problem of "statistical power." It means literally the power a procedure has to discern an effect. It is not unlike the problem of administering a chemical to only fifty rats in an attempt to determine if the odds of killing the rat with the substance are 100 to 1. Those may indeed be the odds, but one cannot be sure because one simply has not tried enough rats; the fifty-first rat might tell the tale.

Zelen's example of "power" involves slips of black and white paper. Supposing, he says, one were to cut up sheets of black and white paper into scraps and toss them into the air, the object of the experiment being to determine whether black papers will bunch together if randomly thrown in the air with white bits of paper when they all hit the floor. If one makes three tosses and sees no bunching, one could only tentatively say that paper slips do not have a tendency to bunch. If one makes a hundred tosses and sees no bunching, one's hunch becomes more likely. But if every biostatistics student in the country conducted the experiment, and not one student saw any bunching effect, then it would be much easier to say definitely that black paper slips have no tendency to bunch. Though one can never be 100% sure.

The number of tosses, or the number of times the experiment is done, and the numbers of slips of paper, or the number of subjects in the experiment, defines the "power" of the study. The more subjects and the more times a statistical experiment is done, the more power the experiment has.

In the Woburn cluster, as with any cluster investigation, the problem was also one of power. All an orthodox statistical study could do, because there were so few leukemia cases, was say that something odd had occurred and that the odds of its having happened by chance alone were 100 to 1. As is said, rare events happen, however rarely.

What Zelen and Lagakos needed was some way of putting the cluster against a wider background. The cluster was odd compared to other leukemia patterns, but Zelen wondered, was it odd against patterns of other disease? Were there other unusual health pictures in Woburn, and did they correlate with the wells? In particular, Zelen and Lagakos wanted to study the pattern of birth defects and reproductive disorders, because these types of illnesses, often genetically based and developing during the vulnerable fetal stage of life, were already suspected of being frequently environmentally related. Substances that could cause birth defects, that is, teratogens, were also often carcinogens. In fact the Council on Environmental Quality had published a report in January of 1981 entitled "Chemical Hazards to Human Reproduction," which concluded, "Although the report is not an exhaustive review of the scientific literature, its findings suggest that the relationship between exposure to chemicals and human reproductive impairment may be an important area of public health concern that deserves more scientific investigation and evaluation."

If there were indeed unusual patterns and they tended to concentrate in areas served by the wells, that would be a kind of corroborative evidence that something was amiss in the East Woburn health scene. For then the leukemia cluster would not be the only freak.

Also, introducing the parameter of birth defects helped avoid another problem—"hypotheses in light of the data," which means an idea occurs to you because some phenomenon has already suggested itself. This can tend to bias a study too in that a scientist does not set out on a pure blind instinct, but because something has grabbed his or her attention. Since no one knew if there was an unusual rate of birth defects or not in Woburn, this dimension of the study provided the chance to look for something not already known to be there.

But how to add to the subjects of study? How, in other words, to survey enough nooks and crannies?

For a Cleaner Environment (FACE) provided the solution, for if FACE could provide people power, then

Zelen's department could provide statistical power.

The idea of a collaboration between the department of biostatistics and FACE evolved, as Zelen and Lagakos had the idea of administering telephone questionnaires to a cross section of all Woburn residents to determine whether households had experienced health effects such as miscarriages, low birth weight, spontaneous abortion, or birth defects, and other childhood illnesses.

FACE volunteers would make the phone calls hoping to reach a target population of approximately 10,000 residents. And Zelen's team would analyze the results biostatistically, using the computer services at the Dana-Farber Cancer Institute of the Harvard Medical School. In fact, Zelen succeeded in convincing the institute to donate the computer time, without which the study would not have been conceivable. There would not have been a way for Zelen's department to undertake the Woburn study if it had had to provide or raise the money to conduct the sophisticated analysis of the data it had in mind. The contributions in kind enabled the study of Woburn to take an entirely new approach to cluster investigation.

Zelen's was an ambitious plan for a highly unorthodox collaboration on an unprecedented scale. Normally academic scientists do not rely on layperson help for collecting data. And even with Harvard designing the questionnaire and training the interviewers in how to objectively pose questions, Zelen was aware that "bias," anathema to any scientist, could creep into the process, perhaps as subtly as a change of inflection in the voice of an interviewer on the phone, hinting to the subject that he or she was giving a "right" or "wrong" answer.

Using community volunteers in the first place was risky and largely unprecedented in that ideally only trained epidemiologists will administer epidemiological questionnaires precisely to avoid the odds of creeping, even unconscious bias. But volunteer person power was all that was available, and a study large enough to discern subtle effects needed as much person power as it could have. It was a compromise Zelen and Lagakos made in order to make the study possible, confident their training procedures and the volunteers' own commitment to a truthful, useful study would prevent bias problems.

Zelen and Lagakos too were subject to bias, and so they attempted to drop a Gardol shield down between their methods and their personal interest in the problem. The notion that wells G and H were the bad guys had to be scrubbed from their consciousness and from the consciousness of all the volunteers. That a cluster had been found had also to be put out of everyone's minds. For purposes of the Harvard study, the search was supposed to be starting from scratch.

Anonymity for those answering the questions was the first necessity. Harvard broke the Woburn telephone directory into perfectly randomized lists. Since prefix numbers in Woburn are not determined by the geographical location of the phone, a volunteer would receive a list of numbers without having any idea who or where in Woburn he or she was calling. Each household being interviewed was assigned a number, and each volunteer was told to discontinue an interview if the voice on the other end of the telephone line sounded familiar.

Also, Zelen and Lagakos put distance between themselves and the FACE volunteers. Barbara Wesson, a young biostatistics doctoral candidate, became the go-between, coordinating volunteers so that Zelen and Lagakos, those who would ultimately analyze the data, would not develop any conscious or unconscious feelings about any one volunteer that might lead to taking a skewed view of the data when it came time to analyze it. Science and emotion could not mix.

In mounting the study, Zelen by definition was marching his department into new terrain. He was attempting to use biostatistics to hone in where epidemiology and toxicology had the rightful lead, but where, it seemed, neither epidemiology nor toxicology could penetrate further. Both the CDC and the MDPH had done as much in Woburn as they felt could be done. No follow-up studies were under way. But since there was as yet no answer to the question of cause, there remained an opening for science Zelen believed he and his department could fill.

In the meantime the search for cause in Woburn was joined by another unusual partner, one that would become increasingly important in the study of toxic waste—hydrogeology, or the study of underground water and its movements through the earth. While Zelen and his colleagues were hatching a new approach to statistical significance, engineers at the Massachusetts Department of Environmental Quality Engineering (DEQE) were busy literally underground, attempting to determine where the toxic waste and the water were and how and when the two had met.

If the pattern of contamination found by the DEQE, for example, were found to parallel the pattern of disease found by Harvard—bad health appearing when there was bad water—then the Woburn study would have put pieces of the cluster puzzle together in a manner no one had ever tried before.

Robert Cleary, the environmental engineer with the DEQE assigned to Woburn, has an office that is simply a desk among desks set in a row not unlike what one would expect to see on the officers' floor of a great big bank. For an agency that is concerned with the protection of the environment, the physical environment of the agency is sterile and aloof. Cleary, however, is not.

His eyes fill with the curious excitement of a scientist with a tough, enticing nut to crack when he says, "the question which bedeviled us was when did those wells get contaminated and with what."

To find out would require dollars and time of the kind not usually invested in cluster investigations, certainly an unprecedented amount of both. But the inherent drama of the events in Woburn, the publicity it attracted, and the lobbying Anne Anderson and FACE had been doing were beginning to pay off. They had a clear ability to impress public officials with the logic of their arguments, and the simple goal of their efforts: they wanted to know what, if anything, had caused the leukemias. The reasonableness of their intentions was difficult to shunt aside.

One of the first elected officials FACE had approached, Nicholas Paleologos, who had grown up in Woburn, was impressed with the chronicle of Woburn events. And he did not want to see the Woburn investigation end with a question mark. He facilitated what would prove to be an extraordinary commitment to finding an answer in Woburn.

When the DEQE budget came up for discussion in

1980 in the Massachusetts legislature, Paleologos offered a carefully worded amendment from the floor that would incorporate into the budget $100,000 to DEQE specifically for the "administration of a program to test the air and water in the Woburn Industri-Plex area for the purpose of determining if a connection exists between the hazardous waste deposits and abnormally high incidence of cancer in that geographical area." It was no small matter, but it hung on a single word—*connection.* If epidemiology shied away from the word *link,* here was a different umbrella under which DEQE could begin tracing back from the heads of wells G and H to discover the source of the toxic contamination.

About this same time, FACE had been active at the federal level as well. Bruce Young and Anne Anderson's testimony in the summer of 1980 had focused Congress on the relevance of Superfund to the well-being of individuals.

The Industri-Plex site had already been designated for clean-up funds under Superfund, but then largely through the efforts of federal representatives of the Woburn area, Edward M. Kennedy in the Senate, and Edward Markey in the House of Representatives, wells G and H were designated Superfund sites as well. Even though the wells had been shut off, the aquifer remained contaminated and before attempts could be made to clean it, if any could be made, the extent of the contamination had to be determined. Richard Leighton of the federal EPA regional office in Boston was assigned to the Woburn projects: both G and H wells and the Industri-Plex site.

The combined forces of Leighton and Cleary and con-

sulting engineers retained to work with them jumped
Woburn up onto a new level of cluster investigation as
far as hunting for physical evidence was concerned. No
one had ever looked into aquifers in this detail before
in connection with a cluster of illness involving deaths.
Indeed, the idea of attempting to establish the history
of an aquifer that would go back at least twenty years
was practically unheard of in connection with such a
cluster.

But peering into the underground is not a matter of
sinking the geoscope down into the earth and having a
look. Tracing underground contamination is a painstaking matter in which progress is measurable in feet
per year.

The search begins with what is called "groundwater
modeling," the technique of determining the movement
of water underground. But to arrive at such a profile,
one must first understand the underground layers of
earth in the area in question, for what those layers consist of—sand, shale, rock—determines how fast water
travels. So, to know in what direction water is moving
and how fast, one has to determine through what type
of layers of earth the water must move.

After studying the logs and records of the drillers who
had originally dug wells G and H, as well as records
pertaining to other wells in Woburn, the engineers concluded that wells G and H drew on a "recharging" underground area a maximum of 10 miles square. This
therefore was the huge pie from which they had to carve
manageable pieces to study. And at first the assumption
was that contamination of G and H wells had originated
around the Industri-Plex site.

The engineers used a technique called seismic refraction, which had been developed to help locate oil deposits underground. The concept depends on the fact that sound waves travel at different speeds and directions, depending on what they hit—oil, water, or a layer of the earth. The waves may bounce or be deflected, depending on the density of the various strata, and so it is a way of seeing by learning what is in the way of the waves. In Woburn, the idea was not of course to find oil but to determine where the water was and what it met on its travels that would affect its direction and speed of flow.

Cleary, Leighton, and their colleagues sank iron rods and test pipes into the contaminated ground to mark grids in the larger pie. When seismic refraction is used, small explosions are detonated at one end of a grid to produce sound waves. These then reach a geophone, a microphone for listening underground, placed at the opposite end of the section, which is attached to a stylus recorder like the type used to draw the human heartbeat in electrocardiograms. As the sound waves encounter the varying densities of the earth, the recorder pen squiggles accordingly, in effect printing out the structure of the earth as if it were a layer cake. Sound wave squiggles reproduce the earth pattern necessary to determine how fast water or contamination move.

Cleary and Leighton set up a field office in a trailer at Industri-Plex just outside the Cyclone fencing they had themselves installed to mark the boundaries of the waste site when money to do the job was slow to come from Superfund.

While the wind caught breezes and set their flag markers fluttering, the engineers worked, sometimes setting a dynamite charge to see what it recorded, and sometimes simply hitting a heavy hammer to a metal plate to achieve the same sound effect.

As this work was going on, but totally independent of it, design and planning of the Harvard questionnaire study was under way. Thus the mystery of the Woburn leukemia cluster was being approached from two separate, but equal, fronts, which would, if they ultimately came together, begin to shape a new multidimensional kind of epidemiology.

The Harvard study questionnaire sought to gather information from randomly selected Woburn residents who had lived in Woburn since 1960 about their medical histories. Volunteers, 301 of them, coordinated by FACE, received an orientation briefing from the Harvard staff and were instructed to use a pleasant, polite telephone manner, not to interrupt households by calling at dinner time, and to maintain objectivity at all times, sticking to the prewritten questions as though to a script and not enhancing or embellishing the conversation with any personal opinion. Except for the fact that its announced purpose was to try to answer "some unresolved question about the impact of hazardous waste on health"—a tip of the hand the study could have done without—the questionnaire contains no subjective word. It is purely a tool for gathering facts.

The questionnaire, eleven pages long, asked the interviewees about the size of the household, ages and dates of birth of each person in it, whether or not persons in the household had suffered miscarriages or stillbirths, whether anyone in the household suffered from anemia

or other blood diseases, birth defects, or genetic conditions, cancer, diabetes, heart or blood pressure problems, infertility, kidney problems, learning disabilities,
lung or respiratory problems, neurologic or nervous system problems, skin problem or allergies, serious digestive problems such as ulcers, or other serious conditions
such as blindness and deafness. Though the questionnaire asked the interviewee to include illnesses only if
they had been medically diagnosed, that is, confirmed
by a doctor, the questionnaire did not provide defini-
tions of these illnesses either to the interviewer or interviewee. So such terms as "genetic conditions" were
left to the interviewee to determine. But once the interviewee answered "yes" to any question, the interviewer
then asked him or her to be as specific as possible about
the disease, to, for example, name which type of cancer
had been diagnosed in the family.

The study aimed to reach a random sample equal to
roughly 70% of the Woburn population that had tele-
phones. FACE went about the business of recruiting volunteers to begin making the calls. Each volunteer was
supposed to be responsible for twenty-five calls; not
everyone made the quota. Some volunteers made over
100 calls each.

Starting in April 1982 the volunteers received computer printout sheets that listed the telephone numbers
for which each would be responsible. The lists represented segments of a larger random sample of the town,
random meaning each household in Woburn had as good
a chance as any other to be included. The sample had
been culled in such a way as to ensure that no matter
how many phone calls were actually made, a cross section of the entire town would have been sampled.

In some ways the procedure was crude. The study questionnaire, though designed by statistical experts with advice from a physician, amounted to door-to-door epidemiology done on the telephone.

It is somewhat ironic then that this apparently simply styled procedure constituted a landmark effort in the epidemiology of leukemia clusters. Virtually all other investigations had stopped at demonstrating statistical significance and usually concluded by saying no conclusions could be drawn, adding, by way of finding comfort perhaps, that cluster investigations generally ended inconclusively.

The study undertaken by Harvard's biostatistics department had the potential to break this frustrating cycle, because through the use of volunteers a lot of data would be collected, and they would be subjected to vigorous biostatistical analysis by Zelen and his team, highly regarded as experts in the analytical procedures necessary.

Zelen was excited by the prospect of the Woburn study, although he did not discuss the work publicly very much. In fact, in October 1983 the *Boston Globe Sunday Magazine* published an article that cast Zelen as somewhat obsessed by the possibilities of his study. It said of Zelen, "He is determined, colleagues say, to 'crack Woburn.' "

But Zelen knew, as would anyone familiar with the limits of any sort of epidemiology, that even his study could not "prove" cause and effect. It could just come closer.

Telephone surveying continued through September 1982, and computer analysis of the data began in 1983. In the meantime the Massachusetts DEQE was proceeding with its underground water studies. Using the seismic refraction techniques in the grid pattern, engineers worked away at the 10-square-mile area, grid by grid, back from the G and H well heads, in an attempt to discover the source of contamination.

Their profile also included taking a look at the geological structure, and it became clear that the bedrock in the 10-square-mile area sloped in a southwesterly direction, with much of the bedrock area, according to the geological survey report, "dominated by a north-south trending trench with the rock surface rising rapidly to the east and west." The trench is somewhat like an underground bowl, and, it turned out, wells G and H reached into the deepest part of the trench, the precise location where any contamination underground would tend to collect. In other words, it became clear that wells G and H had been placed at perhaps the worst possible position with respect to the land's underground structure and probably should not have been dug there in the first place. In fact, when the wells were being dug in the 1960s, no review of the geology was made. The task at hand was to find water, and engineers at the time knew only that the Aberjona River Valley, swampy and marshy as it was, was a source of abundant water. And the area was one of the few left in Woburn free of development and open enough to meet the state requirements that all municipal water be surrounded by open area to avoid what was then considered the threat to groundwater—contamination from sewer and septic systems. Unfortunately, abundance and openness did not ensure quality of the water.

Some of the sample wells sunk by the DEQE engineers here and there throughout the grid area also were contaminated with the chemicals found in wells G and H, and the engineers worked bit by bit, poking into the ground following the plume of contamination, moving on, poking again, in a process not unlike poking into a rotting peach here and there to see how far the rot extends.

Slowly the underground portrait emerged. For one thing, the engineers learned that wells G and H did not draw water from the Aberjona River, as had been assumed, but that in fact perhaps the river drew some of the underground water that fed the wells. Also, it became clear that the contamination plumes were consistently "bottom seeking," that is, heading almost directly toward the bottom of the bowl, namely, the feeding pools of wells G and H. The research also began to show that the plumes were traveling from a point north and northeast of the wells but not as far as the core of the Industri-Plex site. In fact, to the surprise of almost all concerned, it began to look like toxics from the mammoth waste site were not headed toward G and H at all.

Instead, G and H contamination seemed to emanate from several other ongoing industrial operations.

In March of 1982 the consulting engineers and the EPA released a report entitled "Chlorinated Solvent Contamination of the Groundwater in East Central Woburn, Mass." The report suggested that groundwater flowed toward wells G and H *not* from the huge Industri-Plex site but from an area near the industrial operation owned by the W. R. Grace Company and operated as its Cyrovac Division. Groundwater flowing under this property would flow in a southwesterly direction, directly toward wells G and H, and so would surface water like the runoff from rain since it too would be carried southwesterly due to the direction of the land's drainage. And toxic contaminants, including TCE, were found in test wells subsequently sunk on the Cyrovac site.

Contaminants including TCE were also found in test wells located on the property of the J. J. Riley Company, the tannery on Salem Street in East Woburn that had been in operation for decades and that had been purchased by the Beatrice Foods Company in 1978. No contamination was found in groundwater upstream from these two properties, only below them.

In May of 1982, making use of the groundwater studies, eleven Woburn families, including Anne Anderson, Donna Robbins, Pat and Michael Zona, Richard and Mary Toomey, and Kevin and Patricia Kane, filed a civil suit against the Grace Company and Beatrice Foods, leaving an "et al." on the list of defendants to accommodate others who might later be named as additional information became available. The complaint said that poor waste disposal practices by the defendant companies led to groundwater contamination, which in turn had led to fatal illnesses in their families.

Both Grace and Beatrice denied any involvement in the water contamination, and in November of 1982 the Grace Company filed a motion to dismiss the case citing Rule 11 of the Federal Civil Code. Judge Walter Jay Skinner, who considered the Grace motion, noted that indeed this rule could be a "useful tool to restrain frivolous and abusive litigation." However, he denied the motion to dismiss the case on January 24, 1983, stating that although the Woburn families did not have "conclusive" proof that groundwater contamination had caused the leukemias, laboratory data on the effects of TCE and statistical data on the increased incidence of leukemia provided a "sufficient basis for a good faith" attempt to find remedy in civil court. Through 1983, attorneys for both plaintiffs and defendants began gathering evidence and preparing their respective cases. The long arm of Woburn had reached the law.

12

Toxic Tort and the Limits of Proof

IN MATTERS WHERE the science of cause lags behind the signs of effect, the vacuum of time is filled by the legal system: judges, lawyers, and juries. Legal cases involving injuries or damages believed to be related to the toxic waste problem have become part of a body of law known as "toxic tort," which grew out of law applied traditionally to consumer product safety. In consumer tort, or injury law, if a consumer is injured by a product shown to be faulty and negligently designed, the consumer can seek compensation from the manufacturer of the product, and the two parties slug it out in court in much the same way as parties battle over the proverbial broken sidewalk.

But in matters of toxic waste and its potential relationship to human disease, evidence, proof, and responsibility are slippery concepts rendering toxic tort law slippery as well. Plaintiffs can be a few individuals, neighbors, or whole towns and communities; hundreds of people can join in one enormous class action. Often the stakes can reach into billions of dollars.

As Dr. Irving Selikoff, the scientist most closely associated with research on asbestos and health, remarked to a gathering of attorneys at a conference in Rochester, New York, in October 1984, "while some people on hearing the words *toxic tort* might ask what bakery to go to to get one, others know this legislation is of growing national interest, one in which evenhandedness is not so easy to come by."

The idea of there being a civil legal remedy or financial compensation from injury related to toxic wastes derived from the turn-of-the-century awareness that workers might suffer on-the-job injury and that the industrial revolution carried with it some burden, particularly on the part of employers, to compensate employees for the new kind of dangers they faced or damages they incurred while working.

Because the potential impact of toxic material on human health was not widely appreciated until the late 1970s, legal suits over toxic materials filed earlier than that tended to focus on damages to property. For example, in 1964 fumes and particles from an aluminum reduction plant contaminated a cattle ranch, and the owner received compensation for nuisance, defined as "an activity which significantly interferes with the plaintiff's use and enjoyment of property." The same aluminum plant also caused some gases to settle on the rancher's property, making the plant also liable for "trespass," namely the intentional discharge of material it should have known would be harmful in a way that would "invade the plaintiff's property and the exclusive possession thereof."

An early case involving a chemical effect on human health was decided in 1848 in favor of a worker, Malitovsky, who was compensated for a burn he suffered due to a defective chemical drum. He won the case on the grounds that his employer was "negligent," that is, guilty of conduct that "falls below the standard established by law for the protection of others against unreasonable risk of harm."

The principles of nuisance, trespass, negligence, as well as the idea of strict liability, namely, that someone who carries on "abnormally dangerous activity" is liable for ensuing harm even if he or she exercises care to prevent the harm, are the foundation of the common law tort system, wherein a citizen can seek compensation for the improper actions of another.

But where toxic waste and public health are concerned, pinning the blame can be especially tricky business. The proof of the link between any given toxic substance and cancer, for example, may still be incubating in the laboratory as scientists attempt to solve the mysteries of DNA. In a court of law, proof need not be irrefutable, though irrefutability helps. What matters in civil court is a "preponderance" of the evidence, literally how much evidence is needed to tip the scale of justice in favor of one side or the other.

Proof becomes a matter of degree; how much is enough to hold sway. But legal proof and scientific proof are of basically different nature. Epidemiologists and biologists speak of "probabilities," while lawyers prefer "likelihoods." As Professor Neil Orloff of the Cornell University Center for Law Research, who has studied the working of "preponderance of the evidence" standard of the law, says "epidemiologists are unable to prove causation; they can only show associations . . . so you put layer of association upon association in the hope that you produce enough proof."

Orloff observes, "Toxic tort is a very crude system that results in these complex issues going to court . . . the legal system finesses the complex scientific issues by sending them to a jury to let the jury decide."

There are a number of basic problems, apart from proving cause and effect, to cope with when the standards of toxic tort law are applied to toxic waste. For one thing, there is the matter of the statute of limitations: If a toxic exposure causes a cancer, it may not do so for decades, and a victim might not become aware of an injury until many years too late to file a claim. There is also the problem of identifying the villains. Most waste sites—Woburn's included—are a veritable brew of chemicals with a melange of ownership, so it is difficult to know who was responsible for the dumping of what when. And "midnight dumpers," those who abandon waste any old place, like the dumpers who left the barrels of polyurethane near the Aberjona River in 1979, which triggered the sampling of wells G and H, do not leave a note advising potential victims whom to sue. Also, victims may be difficult to identify. Jimmy Anderson, unfortunately, was suffering a clearly identifiable disease. But are victims only those who have already died, or also those who may die, or who may suffer only recurring headaches or nausea from something like the "Woburn smell"?

Finally there is the matter of cost and meeting the burden of proof. Normally the plaintiff has the burden of proving that some harm was done, which in a toxic tort case can mean accumulating documents and deeds and scientific reports and expert testimony and literally thousands of dollars of lawyers' time. Ordinary people usually do not have the financial resources to bring a toxic tort claim, and so many cases are brought to court on a contingency basis by lawyers who invest the costs and deduct them and professional fees from settlements or verdicts in the plaintiffs' favor. Roughly one third of all dollars awarded to injured parties under product liability law, for example, are paid to the lawyers who handle the cases.

Out-of-court settlement funds are a relatively neat way to "dispose of," to use a preferred attorney term, large and potentially protracted litigation. Merrell Dow Pharmaceuticals, for example, in July 1984 established a $120 million fund, to be paid over twenty years, to approximately 700 women who claimed that, as a result of their having taken the drug Bendectin to control nausea during pregnancy, their children suffered birth defects.

But the most famous toxic tort settlement, perhaps a contributing precedent of the Bendectin settlement, came earlier that year on the eve of trial in Brooklyn, New York, in connection with the infamous defoliant Agent Orange. The suit had been five years in the making and, as a class action suit, embraced up to 100,000 Vietnam War veterans who claimed exposure to the defoliant used during the war had led to illness among them—including cancers, skin disease, and birth defects in their children. They claimed Agent Orange had been contaminated during the manufacturing process by highly toxic and carcinogenic dioxin by-products.

Seven companies, including Dow Pharmaceuticals,

who produced the chemicals, were named as defendants, as was the federal government, which could be held responsible for injuries to nonmilitary personnel, since military veterans cannot sue for war-related injuries. The case exemplified a variation on liability law—the concept of alternative liability—which holds that a defendant need not prove specifically who caused the damage if several plaintiffs may have been involved. This concept developed from a case called *Summers v. Tice*, decided in California in 1948. In this case two quail hunters fired negligently at the plaintiff Summers, but only one shot hit him in the eye. He could not establish which hunter had fired the damaging shot, so the presiding judge switched the burden of proof to the hunters, necessitating that they demonstrate they had not caused the injury. Since neither hunter was able to prove the other had done the damage, they were both held liable. In the Agent Orange case it was impossible to determine which chemical company had produced the contaminated batches of Agent Orange, of which about 12 million gallons were used in Vietnam to destroy brush and ground cover.

A few hours before jury selection was about to begin, attorneys in the case announced that the defendant companies, still denying liability, were going to establish a $180 million fund to operate over twenty-five years, to compensate any American, New Zealander, or Australian veteran who could establish any injury to themselves, their wives, or children as a result of their exposure to dioxin. Some 170,000 veterans had filed claims to the fund by the February 1985 deadline.

The key issue here, of course, was establishing the

link between toxic dioxin on the one hand and disease on the other. Like carbon tetrachloride, trichloroethylene, and so many others, the dioxin family of compounds, actually called dibenzo-para-dioxins, is known to be dangerous to humans. They can cause severe acne, or chloracne, in humans as well as acute and fatal poisoning. However, cancer, including the soft cell sarcoma–type suffered by many of the veterans, have been observed only in laboratory animals. Among the veterans it was unclear whether there were "true clusters" of cancer, given the extent of the intervening variables and routine exposures in the lives of the veterans since leaving Vietnam. After the settlement was announced, lawyers said they thought they would have been able to prove a link between dioxin and cancer in about 1,000 cases, and birth defects in less than 1,500 cases. In fact, the claim of Kerry Ryan, who was born in 1971 with a variety of serious birth defects, was denied, even though her parents, Maureen and Michael Ryan of Long Island, New York, had been leading plaintiffs in the Agent Orange suit. The attorneys handling the settlement said it was just too difficult to say within a "preponderance of the evidence standard" that Kerry's multiple health problems were caused by her father's exposure.

What can happen when there is strongly persuasive proof is patently clear in the case of asbestos, which has a more or less unquestioned association with mesothelioma, a rare cancer of the lining of the lungs and intestines, as well as asbestosis, a progressive deterioration of lung function. Legal claims were being filed for personal injuries against asbestos producers, mainly the Johns Manville Corporation, at the rate of roughly 400 per month, and were expected to reach approximately 25,000 by early 1986 and 52,000 by the end of the century. As of August 26, 1982, when the Manville Corporation declared bankruptcy to shield itself from asbestos litigation, some $661 million had been paid in connection with claims that had been settled out of court or awarded by a judge and jury, and Manville had estimated that the asbestos claims against it, including ones yet to be filed, could surpass $2 billion.

In addition, asbestos spawned the first nationwide class action for property damage resulting from a product liability question when in 1984 a federal district judge in Philadelphia approved a class action suit against fifty-five separate asbestos manufacturers brought on behalf of half the primary schools and secondary schools in the United States, since according to the United States Environmental Protection Agency, about 14,000 of the nation's 36,000 public and private schools used asbestos in their ceiling board, piping, insulation, or other corners of their buildings. The United States Department of Education estimated it would cost about $1.1 billion to remove the asbestos, and the Congress of February 1985 had appropriated $50 million for this purpose. By comparison, when the suit was filed, the plaintiffs sought approximately $300 million in damage awards, to mitigate the costs of removing asbestos from the schools, and another approximately $150 million to cover medical monitoring of the population exposed, estimated by the EPA as 15 million children and roughly 1.4 million adult school employees. Given that mesothelioma may take up to thirty years to develop, the children involved would be at risk for many years following settling of the suit.

In an attempt to emerge from bankruptcy protected

against the expected avalanche of asbestos claims, in June 1984 the Manville Corporation proposed to establish a trust fund for asbestos victims, financed by cash, insurance payments, and a dilution of its stock, representing a minimum of $700 million.

To date there have been no toxic tort claims involving a cluster of illness to compare with asbestos in terms of money, although with some 22,000 toxic waste sites discovered in America, the number of potential plaintiffs could climb into the millions. Radiation cases, however, come close to asbestos in terms of the nature of proof. For ionizing radiation, the sort that emanates to some extent from natural background sources such as cosmic rays, as well as the sort used in diagnostic x-rays and nuclear bomb making, testing, and exploding, can induce virtually any form of human cancer, in particular the myelocytic leukemias and acute lymphocytic leukemias.

The national implications of the radiation cases were sharply focused in May of 1984 when Federal District Judge Bruce S. Jenkins, hearing a nine-week trial in Salt Lake City without a jury, ruled that radioactive fallout from above-ground military nuclear bomb tests in the 1950s had caused ten people to die of cancer and that the United States government had been negligent when it failed to warn residents of northern Arizona, southern Utah, and Nevada of the potential effects of the fallout and to advise them on ways to minimize its effects. The testing had been extensive. Between 1945 and June of 1976 the United States detonated 466 of a total of 588 nuclear test bombs in Nevada.

It was a classic example of the complexities of what

happens when epidemiology meets the law, particularly years after the fact. It took Judge Jenkins seventeen months to prepare his 490-page decision. He had to steer between those cases of cancer that could be shown to be "proximately caused" by radiation and those for which links were more elusive. And he had to evaluate contradictory epidemiological evidence, fitting medical and statistical uncertainty, even dispute, into a framework of the law and the concept of the preponderance of the evidence. He had to evaluate the specific cases before him in the context of the general evidence available about the effects of radiation.

There was first a study by Dr. Joseph F. Lyon and others, published in the *New England Journal of Medicine* in February 1979, which found that deaths from leukemia, particularly among ten- to fourteen-year-old children who lived in counties of Utah that experienced high fallout, were about two and a half times higher than rates in the area prior to the testing. And there was a preliminary report by Dr. Glyn G. Caldwell, who had worked on the earliest Woburn investigations, and others at the federal Centers for Disease Control (published in October 1980 in the *Journal of the American Medical Association* [JAMA]) which found that there was a statistically significant increase of deaths from leukemia—a cluster of 9 cases where 3.5 would have been suspected—among 3,224 men who participated in the 1957 nuclear test explosion of the bomb called "Smoky."

There was also a report presented at the trial in 1982 by Dr. Carl J. Johnson (published in *JAMA* in January 1984) which said that a group of 4,125 Mormons who lived in southwestern Utah when tests were conducted in nearby Nevada experienced roughly twice as many deaths from leukemia and thyroid, breast, and gastrointestinal cancer than would have been statistically expected.

Judge Jenkins also heard testimony from residents of the area, who stated that dusts from the test clouds settled all around their homes and after the tests they were told by government officials not to drink locally produced milk or eat local dairy products and even to wear badges to detect bodily radioactive contamination. Jenkins also heard government testimony that tests were postponed when wind direction might have meant the radioactive clouds would blow over the populous Las Vegas and Los Angeles areas, leaving them to travel into rural, sparsely settled Utah, Nevada, and Arizona instead.

But there was evidence on the other side of the scale as well. The Mormon study was hotly contested at trial by witnesses appearing on behalf of the United States. And the Lyon study on childhood leukemias was challenged by Dr. Charles E. Land and others of the Environmental Epidemiology Branch of the National Cancer Institute, who concluded in a paper (published in January 1984 in the journal *Science*) that the rates Lyon had observed seemed higher because the rates prior to the nuclear testing had been "anomalously" low compared to other similar counties in the United States. This "lowness," the Land report suggested, could have been because fewer leukemia cases were reported than existed because of misdiagnosis or poor disease reporting techniques.

Judge Jenkins therefore had to visualize the medical

treatment situation that obtained in remote postwar Utah. There was certainly no tumor registry at the time, and physicians were scarce: in seventeen southern Utah counties, the high fallout areas, there was only one medical board–certified physician to serve roughly 125,000 people. Land and others attributed Lyon's finding essentially to inaccurate record keeping about cancer and concluded "the evidence for an increase in childhood leukemia mortality in southern Utah as a result of exposure to radioactive fallout between 1950 and 1958 appears, on closer examination of available data, to be slight or non-existent."

Then Dr. Caldwell and others of the CDC published a follow-up report on the military men in the Smoky test, which added information about deaths from cancers other than leukemia among the group and reported on nearly the full group of 3,217 male and female test participants.

The leukemia results held; that is, there was still a statistically significant increase of leukemia. But the follow-up report concluded that although deaths from melanoma, cancer of the pharynx, and cancers of the brain, breast, eye, and genital tract were higher than expected, none of the levels was statistically significant, that is, conceivably attributable to a factor other than chance. And, the scientists said, these other cancers, particularly melanoma, had not been observed among survivors of Nagasaki or Hiroshima in elevated numbers. The follow-up paper concluded that in the absence of higher rates of deaths from cancer other than leukemia, the leukemia finds "may be either attributable to chance or the result of an unknown combination of factors." The paper also added that there was support for the military's position that exposure among its men had been "low."

Of course, some were skeptical of the government's case, supported by the studies of the government agencies, the CDC, and the National Cancer Institute, viewing it as an official attempt not only to avoid specific liability in the fallout cases but also to prevent a political reaction that might accompany revelations that the United States government had knowingly put its own citizens at radiation risk so soon after the nuclear devastation in Japan. In fact, at a dinner honoring W. Dale Haralson of Tucson, Arizona, who tried the plaintiff's case, a law professor presenting an award to Haralson for his courage in confronting the government remarked, "where it is a duty to worship the sun, it is pretty sure to be a crime to examine the law of heat."

Judge Jenkins therefore was aswim in science and politics and history and law. But he found at minimum that the United States government had been negligent in its responsibilities. And in deciding the case in favor of the plaintiffs, he wrote "This opinion speaks in terms of 'natural and probable' consequences, 'substantial factors' and 'things more likely than not.' In the pragmatic world of 'fact' the court passes judgment on the probable. Dispute resolution demands rational decision, not perfect knowledge." The judge had put his finger on the very words involved and called attention to their limits. In so doing, he showed that language can be no more precise in describing the scientific facts than the facts themselves, but that in the meantime, some decisions had to be made. A concept of justice would pull the train of environmental health if it could not propel itself. The

Jenkins decision in the case officially called *Allen v. United States* was appealed by the federal government and as of April 1985 awaited final resolution.

The Agent Orange, asbestos, and radiation cases had cousins also making their way through the courts, for it was inevitable that problems of property damage and health effects related to toxic waste sites would join the body of tort law.

The Velsicol case, involving Hardeman County, Tennessee, and residential wells on Toone-Teague road, had, for example, an interesting gestation. Though dumping at the site ceased in 1975, that was not the end of the story. In 1978 tests of the groundwater showed that indeed wastes from the site had so seriously contaminated five wells that their owners were told not to use them anymore for drinking or anything else, leaving forty-seven adults and children without access to usable water. One study of the wells revealed a concentration of 4,800 parts per billion of carbon tetrachloride, a common cleaning solvent, known to be carcinogenic. The level was astronomically high. With their wells no longer available, families in the area had to buy water for use until their homes could be connected to the municipal water system, which would cost about $30,000.

According to the book *Hazardous Waste in America*, the Velsicol Company continued to deny liability, although company representatives did visit the families involved, offering one a $4,000 check and the market value of their house if the family would indemnify Velsicol against further action. Investigators continued, and gradually Velsicol involvement in the contamination became more public. The company paid the hook-up charge so the families could draw from municipal water, and when residents refused to sell their homes, Velsicol replaced the plumbing systems. But then the health consequences of the contamination came into the equation. In November 1978 after public attention had been captured by Love Canal, a University of Cincinnati medical team began a series of examinations of 112 people living or formerly living in the Toone-Teague area. The study found that some residents had enlarged livers—the liver is the prime detoxifying organ of the body—and that many suffered headaches, fatigue, dizziness, eye burning, bloodshot eyes, tingling skin, and muscle weakness.

Faced with both property damage and adverse health effects, residents of the Toone-Teague area of Hardeman County sued the Velsicol Company for $2.5 billion in a class action suit that covered over 100 named defendants. And if, as is possible, the contamination spreads to the deep artesian aquifer, the water supply for the city of Memphis could also be affected. According to the EPA, complete cleanup of the site would cost $165 million.

At St. Louis Park, Minnesota, where the city had found in 1973 it had bought a toxic mess from the Reilly Tar and Creosote Company, which it had agreed to hold harmless, the ensuing litigation involved layer upon layer of involvement, with the city attempting to void its indemnification so it could sue Reilly. The city was joined by the federal government and the local housing authority, which had intended to use the contaminated land.

At Love Canal, medical confusion added to the potential legal confusion as residents, worried and weary from battling to understand if they would be compensated for the property damage to their homes, heard in 1980 first that they had suffered serious chromosomal damage, which could possibly account for the unusual patterns of birth defects in the neighborhood, and then that they had not. The first study had been announced by the EPA, then criticized by other members of the scientific community.

As late as February 1985, conclusions on the level of chromosomal damage had flip-flopped again. By then too, suits filed totaled some $16 billion, although about 1,300 former residents had opted to accept settlements ranging from $2,000 to $400,000 each to cover property damage and medical claims. The settlements were paid from a $20 million fund of which the Hooker Chemical Company, continuing to deny liability, paid $6 million. The balance was paid into the fund by Hooker's insurance company and Niagara Falls City and School Board. One million dollars was set aside to cover health costs that may in future be ascribed to the site, but approximately ninety former Love Canal residents refused to take part in the settlement, preferring to take their chances in court in the tort system.

In Jackson Township, New Jersey, in November 1983, toxic tort law was nudged a little further in a decision awarding $17.6 million dollars to ninety-seven families, including James McCarthy, who had testified along with Anne Anderson and Bruce Young at congressional hearings on waste sites in June of 1980.

In the case of the town's landfill, which took five years

to get to court, the jury found procedures the town had used to operate the landfill had been faulty and contributed to contamination of the water supply with chemicals, including TCE, which in turn contributed to the illnesses and deaths, skin rashes, headaches, chronic vaginitis, and so forth among the plaintiffs. Of the $17 million, most of which was to be covered by the town's insurance, $8.2 million was allotted to pay for annual checkups for residents so that warning signs of cancer might be detected. Interestingly the judge instructed the jury that they might find that the plaintiffs suffered from enhanced risk of cancer, not only cancer itself. And also interestingly the jury, while willing to award money for medical costs, emotional distress, and even diminished quality of life, did not award any money to compensate for the loss of property value, the most "provable" of all elements of a toxic tort case involving residents, houses, and groundwater.

Questions of "risk" of cancer are as complicated scientifically as the question of what causes cancer. Mr. McCarthy's nine-month-old daughter Karen died in 1975 of a rare tumor of the kidney, and seven people in eight of the houses nearest the McCarthy's experienced some form of kidney disease.

The "enhanced risk" argument put forth by their lawyers said there was not only the present observable conditions, and others, but also that an "increased susceptibility" to cancer is also a "present condition" in that one is presently physically at higher risk. The arguments rest on being able to prove that toxic chemicals in water ingested by a plaintiff somehow can change the body, without necessarily causing disease at the same time.

In their briefs, lawyers for the plaintiffs argued, among other things, that "compelling consideration of public policy and practicality are responsible for the overwhelming recognition of enhanced risk."

Companies can also be plaintiffs in toxic tort cases, and, for example, in April 1984 a jury awarded the Onan Corporation, which manufactures electric generators and diesel engines in Fridley, a suburb of Minneapolis, Minnesota, $1.5 million of the $6.4 million it sought in claims against the Boise Cascade Corporation, the Burlington Northern Railroad, and the Soo Line Railroad Company. Onan charged that Boise had been responsible for letting toxic creosote escape into the land Onan bought and that the railroads—who were ordered to pay 10% of the total amount awarded—were party to the problem because they carried the hazardous material to the site. Fridley is not far from St. Louis Park, the scene of other creosote troubles.

Even the United States government can be a plaintiff in toxic tort, as evidenced by the *Goliath v. Goliath*–type suit brought in December 1983 for $1.9 billion by the United States Justice Department against the Shell Oil Company, claiming that toxic chemicals such as benzene, vinyl chloride, and the pesticides aldrin and dieldrin were spilled and leaked at a Shell facility located on the grounds of a United States Army arsenal near Denver, contaminating land and water supplies. The army also disposed of waste from chemical weapons production at the arsenal from 1943 to 1969, and Shell announced it would "vigorously oppose the allegations of a Government suit filed against Shell."

The astounding costs, in time and money, that attend

virtually any toxic tort litigation did bring the United States Congress to look for an alternative remedy system when it passed the Comprehensive Environmental Response Compensation and Liability Act, or the Superfund law, in 1980. Partly because it simply did not know what to do about the massive possibilities for litigation that came to light along with the numerous waste sites in the late 1970s and early 1980s, the Congress convened the "301 (e) Study group," named for the section of the law that gave it birth. The group, a panel of twelve lawyers and legal scholars, some in private practice, and representing trial lawyers as well as insurers, were to look into the procedures that applied in litigating toxic waste–related lawsuits.

For a year, the group worked long days, often into the night, according to James R. Zazzali, who served as chairman of the group and who was attorney general for the state of New Jersey at the time. He said "We wouldn't have spent literally thousands of hours if we were attacking the speculation of a problem . . . and we concluded that the available remedies were totally inadequate in the face of maybe as many as 50,000 waste sites."

Professor Frank R. Grad, a talkative and energetic scholar and director of the Legislative Drafting Research Fund at Columbia University's School of Law in New York City, served as reporter for the study group. He distilled his colleagues' opinions and ideas into a written document, which when bound amounted to two volumes, each an inch thick. Grad, while aware that money cannot be paid out indiscriminately, was mindful throughout the work of the study group of the tight interplay between evidence, dollars, and value judgments. Grad easily framed a basic problem: "Even if you can establish liability, you may still have real trouble in terms of fixing damages . . . there is not only the cost of treating an illness such as leukemia, but also the question of how do you value and repay the loss of life, even the loss of wellness?"

The dilemma posed by this elusive variable was alluded to during congressional hearings on the workings of Superfund in 1984 by the then administrator of the Environmental Protection Agency, William D. Ruckelshaus. While characterizing victims of toxic chemicals as "sympathetic people," he also said, "where a person has had some exposure to toxic chemicals, whether at work or through the environment, it is not unexpected that some might draw a connection between the exposure and injury or disease, irrespective of whether science would support such a link. When and how to make compensation poses a serious question of social justice."

The federal government Office of Management and Budget (OMB) has its particular view of the matter as well. And Michael J. Horowitz, general counsel to the OMB, told *Fortune* magazine in November 1983, "I know of no greater fiscal threat for the nineties than the whole question of toxic torts and victims' compensation." In a later memo urging the formation of a cabinet-level group to ride herd on the toxic tort issue, the OMB elaborated its fears and said, in part, "current toxic substances compensation debates replicate the 1970-era debates over social welfare entitlements." These, the memo said, were "created with low initial costs, understated long-term cost estimates, and no appreciation for expansionary pressures being set in motion. Today we are paying for the consequences of 'small' steps taken without understanding of long-term policy and fiscal implications." During the spring of 1985 when reauthorization debate for the Superfund began in earnest once again, the question of victims' compensation still had not been steered to resolution.

Given the traditional epidemiological model and the time lag inherent therein, the issue of appropriate and fair compensation to victims of exposure to toxic wastes would seem to require the reconciliation of distinctly differing points of view. While proof of cause is the goal of law, in some ways it is irrelevant to the practice of medicine. Medicine, as Dr. Irving Selikoff pointed out to the attorneys in Rochester, "begins with human sympathy and the wish to heal," and proof of cause is not always necessary for that. He observed that "causation is the final stage in medicine."

On the matter of providing lawyers food for thought, Selikoff believed "science has been productive." But he added, "as to how you get the science into the courtroom—on that I wish you luck."

13

Unwelcome Vindication

ON JANUARY 18, 1984, snow fell heavily on the sidewalks of Main Street in Woburn, and pedestrians crunched along, hoping to beat the blizzard home before dark. But that evening at the FACE office all lights were lit, and steam condensed on the window as the office heat fought against the cold outside. A handful of FACE members had decided to hold their regular bimonthly meeting despite the weather, sweetening the occasion by buying themselves a chocolate loaf cake.

The business was mixed. There were ordinary announcements standard in any group and a reading of the minutes of the meeting before. There was a discussion of which FACE members would be attending an imminent toxic waste conference in New Hampshire and who would drive. There was the news of a marathon race that a young local Woburn man, Kevin Mahoney, was planning to run on behalf of children who had died of leukemia in Woburn. And the group reviewed an ongoing project to collect hazardous materials found routinely in the home—caustic cleaning agents and solvents and so forth—as a means of calling attention to the common use of materials that can be dangerous.

But despite the ample agenda, there were two un-

237

spoken focal points of the evening. One was the knowledge that in just a few weeks results of the Harvard Biostatistics Department health study would be released. The FACE group could talk only peripherally about the study, for there had been a tight security lid on the analysis of the questionnaires, and even the FACE members closest to the research had no idea what the study had found.

The somewhat excited anticipation had its counterweight, however, for also palpable in the room was the awareness that the night was the third anniversary of Jimmy Anderson's death. Anne Anderson participated actively in the meeting, even laughing at some jokes about the quality of the cake, but her eyes remained full of fresh communicable sadness.

The next day at the Harvard School of Public Health, Marvin Zelen, chairman of the biostatistics department, Steven Lagakos, and Barbara Wesson, who had coordinated the volunteers, talked generally about their work, holding fastidiously to their secrecy rule about the specifics of their findings. They wanted to keep to their promise that the Woburn community would be first to hear the results. But they had also been stung by the comments in the *Boston Globe Magazine* that had characterized them, Zelen in particular, as somewhat crusading know-it-alls who wanted to bring the exceptional prestige and talent of their university to bear on the problem.

So the group was reluctant to talk further to any media person, particularly on the eve of the announcement of their results. But they did, skirting any discussion of findings in favor of a detailed description of the analytical principles involved in the work.

The group seemed extremely mindful of the inherent shortcomings of statistical analyses of clusters and of the stone wall that epidemiological cluster investigations inevitably reach. They spent a good deal of time describing the problem of statistical "power," of not having a large enough sample, something perhaps fresh on Lagakos's mind after a recent trip to populous China, which, he joked, "in terms of available numbers of people is a biostatistician's dream."

To a statistician, method is all, and it is essential to have all potential limits of the method—and almost every statistical method has a limitation—in mind at all times. Lagakos spoke directly to the main limitation with little hesitation, "In cluster investigations there are bound to be false positives, but also it is certain there are some real clusters with causes happening. Sorting them out is the complication. There is no agreed way to do that."

Zelen's group also elaborated their awareness of the problems of the troublesome "hypotheses developed in light of the data." "The danger," said Zelen, "is that something has come to your attention because it is peculiar, so you go and try to find something to pin it on. But that peculiar event may be going on all over the place and you don't know it. That makes your peculiar event a lot less peculiar, unbeknownst to you." In newspaper terms, it is akin to saying your story is no story. It is dog bites man and not the other way around.

Lagakos continued, "Even the most clustered cluster comes to you because there was evidence that something happened. Statisticians simply cannot quantify that 'leading effect'; you just have to have it mind," meaning that while you are designing your questionnaires, you try as much as possible to control the hypotheses developed in light of the data. Lagakos, Zelen, and Wesson sounded as though they had tried to do so.

But as Zelen added from his seat next to Barbara Wesson on the comfortable sofa, "we knew all this when we started, and there would have been little point in repeating the cluster investigation only to arrive at an answer that said 'yes there is a cluster.' By the time we got involved, we and everybody else already knew that.

"So the task became one of looking further and deciding what other kinds of information we should get." The birth defects information had been one additional kind of information, but after the Harvard study had already been planned and under way, an entirely new ingredient became available to the Zelen team to add to their biostatistical mixture. In connection with its work on the underground profile and the tracking of the movement of underground contamination, the Department of Environmental Quality Engineering (DEQE) had also been working on a theoretical computer model that showed how G and H water distributed through Woburn. It was an experimental sort of hydroarchaeology that enabled the engineers to reconstruct how much water surged through the municipal pipes and where it ended up.

When Zelen and Lagakos heard that the water model was being prepared, they were even more intrigued with the possibilities of their study than they had been at the beginning.

It was this water model that had really enabled the Harvard biostatistics study to break away from the pack on investigations of Woburn. The model meant that to the geographical pattern and statistical incidence of leukemia, birth defects, and other disease, Zelen and Lagakos could now apply another overleaf on the map of Woburn—the overleaf of where the contaminated water went and which households were most exposed to it.

If this had been the case of the empty cookie jar, the water model was the equivalent of having found a trail of crumbs.

Lagakos freely admitted that it was the data on exposure to the well water compared to the incidence of the disease which made the Harvard study even more significant than it would otherwise have been.

And although it was no secret that the DEQE and the EPA had been developing the model, it was Zelen's team that had the idea to use the model to see if there was any relationship between where the water went and where children with leukemia lived. Any other institution could have done that too, but did not.

Despite all the fairly detailed talk about method, the Harvard biostatistics team remained tight-lipped about their findings. All Zelen would say was to predict what he thought would be said about the study once the results were in. "If you come out with something that indicates there are health effects additional to the leukemias, people are likely to criticize your methods or say no cause-and-effect relationship had been shown and that there is only an association. If you come out with no association, some people will criticize you by saying that you looked at the wrong diseases and that your exposure data was too gross. So whichever way you come out, people with authority and fervor argue either way." It seemed a pessimistic but realistic appraisal of what reception the study might receive, but it also underestimated what would eventually unfold.

In the meantime with Woburn waiting for its announcement, residents in the nearby town of Lowell received their own bit of news. On January 20, 1984, Dr. David Ozonoff, a physician turned epidemiologist and chief of the Environmental Health Section of the Boston University School of Public Health, announced the results of a study he and colleagues had conducted during 1983 in Lowell. The town, not far from Woburn, had been the home of the Silresim Chemical Corporation, which had operated a toxic waste recycling business but had apparently failed to use proper waste handling procedures. Silresim had gone bankrupt and moved from Lowell.

When authorities investigated the Silresim site after residents complained of smells and that their children could light the ground with a match, they found the soil had been contaminated with chemicals such as benzene and toluene. Though most waste had been removed from the site, the ground remained contaminated, and chemicals volatilized into the air. Drinking water in the area came from the municipal system rather than the groundwater aquifer.

Residents, nevertheless, were worried that the contamination had or would affect their health, and the Massachusetts DEQE contracted with Boston University to investigate the situation. The study, which surveyed approximately 2,000 adults and 1,000 children then resident in Lowell by telephone using Boston University survey staff, found that at Lowell the main source of contamination would have been in the air, causing smells that the study said, "exceeded the sensory threshold."

The study had also found that residents near the site did not experience a higher rate of cancer, stillbirths, miscarriages, or birth defects. On the other hand, the study did find that the closer residents lived to the site, the more they reported feeling respiratory illness like wheezing, tightness in the chest, coughs, persistent colds, and so forth. Though the illness seemed to be related to a resident's proximity to the site, the illnesses reported were not grave. The *Boston Globe* carried the Silresim study press conference on page 15, the first page of its metro region entertainment section, with a rather mixed headline. In bold print the paper said, "Higher rate of ills near toxic site." In lesser print the paper said, "Study uncertain on link to closed plant in Lowell."

The results of the Boston University study did not necessarily relieve the residents, however. According to the *Globe* report on the public meeting held at Lowell City Hall, residents were irritated that the study did not conclusively link their health problems to the site, because the exposure levels detected at the site were extremely low. On the other hand, the study did say "the observed effects seem to be out of proportion to the apparent exposure." One former Lowell resident who declared she had $4,000 in medical bills still to pay for family illnesses she blamed on the site, boldly challenged the study's conclusion, saying "since we moved out we have not had one ear infection, not one cold, not one case of bleeding, no bronchitis, zip. Tell me that is coincidence."

The study was perceived by some as a hedge, or a study that "did not find anything." But Ozonoff believed that the "gradient of complaints"—the closer people lived to the site, the more likely they were to have had health problems—was a significant finding. This was an association of sorts, but it was not perceived as a link. The Silresim study sank from the news like a rock in the sea.

By February 7, 1984, the Boston area was enjoying a warm thaw. That night the Zelen team called together the FACE volunteers and, at last, revealed the study findings but still asked that secrecy prevail until the public meeting scheduled for the next evening at Trinity Church in Woburn. FACE members agreed to oblige.

For her part, Anne Anderson was nowhere to be found for hours prior to the public meeting on February 8, not that she would have leaked the news. On the day that the nation was going to hear the results of an important study that could explain what caused the death of her son, she had had to spend an intense eight hours with her attorney working out the details of her divorce from his father.

As the hour for the meeting and the public announcement approached, it became increasingly difficult to keep the findings secret, however. There were at least a dozen newspaper reporters, as well as correspondents from local and national television and radio, milling around the large church kitchen.They pressed the wall of secrecy anywhere they could in the hope of finding a soft spot, and when one person would not talk, the press moved on in the search of a person who would.

Increasingly it was obvious that the Harvard report

had indeed unearthed something. Here and there were murmurs that the "wells had done it," or "it was the water after all."

Anne Anderson too was standing around the kitchen, helping to make an urn of coffee in between trying to dodge constant questions from reporters and television anchor people trying to get her to talk about how it felt to be vindicated.

When a television anchorperson who had somehow gotten a look at a copy of the Harvard report asked her to tape a preannouncement interview that could be used just as the news was actually being announced before the audience in Woburn, it seemed absurd to hold back any longer, and Anne Anderson consented to talk. By then the results were anyway being freely discussed in the kitchen, with Jan Schlichtmann, the attorney representing the Woburn plaintiffs who had a few days before been very cautious about discussing whether he would want to see a biostatistical study admitted as evidence in the case, now saying that the report certainly would have an important effect on the litigation.

But in all this excitement, Anne Anderson seemed withdrawn. The meeting was a haunting echo of the ambivalence that had been wracking her since Jimmy's diagnosis. If she were right, then it meant his death had been something that could have been prevented. Against such a fact, vindication was a gift of dubious comfort. This point seemed lost in the throng of well-wishers, as the kitchen presented the strange sensation of a party held at a funeral. Anne Anderson took some relief from the crowd in the narrow corridor leading from the kitchen to Bruce Young's office.

There she took a breath, shut her eyes, and leaned her head back against the stone cold cinder block wall. When she was interrupted, nevertheless, she smiled and said, "I'm sorry. I have been emotional before, but never more than I am feeling right now."

And then she spoke the words she had been harboring for fourteen years. "It is devastating news because it stinks. And it is almost more devastating to know it was the wells than if they had nothing to do with it. It means this did not have to happen."

Inside Walker Community Hall, Marvin Zelen was calling things to order. The hall, where in 1979 about twenty strangers gathered to compare amateur notes on childhood leukemia, was now full to folding chair capacity of 250, with some spectators sitting on the linoleum tile floor and crowded in the kitchen, aisles, and stairwells. Seated behind a long folding table on the stage bathed in bright TV lights were Bruce Young, Zelen, Lagakos, and Barbara Wesson, along with Anne Desmond-Sweetser, then president of FACE, who did not have a child with leukemia but who had helped coordinate the volunteers with Wesson.

Anne Anderson found a place along the side wall, standing with Nicholas Paleologos and Donna Robbins. The Toomeys sat in the audience as did the Kanes, including Kevin. Bob Cleary and Rick Leighton attended. Senator Kennedy sent a representative and a written statement. John Truman stood alone in the back of the room. The new mayor of Woburn attended; the former mayor did not.

Others in the audience were ordinary Woburn residents with no particular stake in the leukemia cluster.

One mother and daughter had come out of curiosity, they said, and because the daughter was now a student at the Harvard School of Public Health. The young woman had been born in the apartment where Donna Robbins now lived. Then the family had moved out of Woburn. "Maybe we moved just in time," said the mother, putting her arm around her daughter's shoulder.

Steven Lagakos spoke into a bank of microphones that looked like giraffes each trying to reach higher than the next. There was no other sound in the room as he summarized the study results, filling out for the public in clear precise language the rumors that had been in the air all evening. The study found, he said:

- A consistent pattern of positive associations between the availability of water from wells G and H and the incidence of childhood leukemia, stillbirths, sudden infant deaths, and some birth defects such as cleft palate and Down's syndrome.
- Children with leukemia had on average 21.2% of their yearly water supply coming from the wells compared with 9.5% among those without leukemia.
- The chance of observing a difference this large if there were no link between the well water and leukemia risk was one in fifty.

Lagakos roundly thanked the DEQE for providing the statistical model that had made the study unique. Marvin Zelen made some observations about the "internal consistencies" in the study, namely that birth defects and some other illnesses seemed also to coordinate with smoking patterns among women.

Lagakos then, almost as an afterthought it seemed, mentioned four new cases of leukemia, that is, cases diagnosed since 1980, which the study had counted. He admitted that these new cases gave Woburn a continuing leukemia rate that was higher than would be expected, but that it was still too early to see the rate flatten out assuming the wells had been involved, given the latency period for leukemia, and that the new cases occurred among children who had been conceived prior to the closing of the wells.

The answers Harvard provided were clear on some levels, and complicated on others, and they had not served as the final answer for all. Donna Robbins, for example, had learned from the study that although her son Robbie had lived within the cluster area prior to his diagnosis, her house did not receive much of the G and H water. "I don't know what it means," she commented wistfully. "My mother babysat for Robbie at her house every day, and she was in the middle of where the water went."

The public had a lot of other questions about how the statistically sophisticated study had been conducted and what it really said. A woman from Lowell came to the microphone that had been set up in the aisle and congratulated the Harvard staff for doing a study that, unlike the study of the Silresim site, had "found something." But another woman, about forty, and bundled up despite the heat inside, asked almost agonizingly about her child who had been born with a birth defect, "my daughter was disallowed from your study because we moved away from Woburn. If it wasn't the water, does it mean I did this to her?" Donna Robbins murmured quietly to herself, "another one like me."

All around the hall there was reaction, but there was

no celebration despite the obvious sense that a peak at last had been attained. The Kane family sat in a row, and Kevin, who was then thirteen, shrugged the resigned shrug of a man much older. He had been declared cured of leukemia, one of the two children of the original twelve cases to have survived. He said, "I guess if I knew then what I know now, I would have been more angry about getting sick."

His father shrugged too. "What can you say? Years ago it was just Anne Anderson saying it was the water. Now they fill the hall."

Kevin's mother, Pat Kane, ran her fingers through Kevin's now thick hair and said "what can you do with news like this? You just get very angry. If Anne Anderson had not fought the way she did . . . God, she was right."

John Truman stood taller than most observers around him at the very back of the hall, and though not joyed by the news, the scientist in him remained very intrigued. "It certainly seems to point a further finger at those wells and get closer to the cause-and-effect problem we've been talking so much about."

Richard and Mary Toomey sat in the middle of the audience, reflecting on the memory of their son, Patrick, who had died less than two months after Jimmy Anderson and only two years after his diagnosis. "This only confirms something," remarked Mr. Toomey. "It doesn't change anything." Mrs. Toomey's thoughts drifted off to the night Patrick died in her arms as guests were leaving the Toomey home from the mass the parents had had said for Patrick. She said, "some days before he died he told us maybe we ought to have another baby to take his place, and then three months after he died,

I found I was pregnant. Now we have a lovely daughter, Sheila. But that doesn't change anything either."

Her husband took her hand and said, "it just keeps making you sad that so many kids had to die before we could get to this point. Maybe something will come out of this now."

It seemed odd that, with everyone more or less crediting Anne Anderson with having been right all along and having catalyzed the deeper investigation of the Woburn problem, at the public meeting she was acknowledged in no public way whatsoever. She herself in fact had conducted about 125 telephone surveys for the study and made countless other logistical calls. But because she had played no official role in the study other than as an ordinary member of FACE, she stayed very much in the background.

The public emotion came from others—residents who shouted that they wanted to move; and others who urged them to solve the toxic waste problems by staying put and fighting back. Emotion came from Bruce Young, who derided companies for dumping, for lying, and town officials for "putting their heads in the sand," and who in a profound exclamation of gratitude conveyed with no embarrassment whatsoever, said firmly into the microphone, "I thank God for people like Marvin Zelen and his staff for doing what no one else would do."

Some emotion also came quietly from DEQE officials on whose water distribution model the Harvard report had relied. They said that the model had been in draft form when they supplied it to the Zelen team and that they had not known the water model would be the keystone of the Harvard report. Somehow, communication had broken down between institutions on what had proven to be one of the most interesting pieces of research to be done in the most extensive leukemia cluster investigations ever undertaken in the United States.

The next day the *Boston Globe* ran a front page story bannered "Woburn Leukemia Linked to Toxic Waste." And there was no respite for questions for the Zelen team, Bruce Young, Anne Anderson, or any other interested parties media members could locate. And all day long Anne Anderson in particular tried to sidestep the language of vindication that reporters kept trying to put in her mouth.

The Harvard results were being described in the Boston press, and in subsequent national wire stories, as "historic." The biostatistics department was so unprepared for the onslaught of requests for the study, it ran out of copies.

But the initial reaction in the epidemiological community to the biostatistics department results were cautious. A few days after the report was released, Dr. Laurence Garfinkle, vice-president for epidemiology of the American Cancer Society, seemed noncommital. "There have been reports of leukemia clusters in the past. Some have been very unusual. Having a cluster in a particular area is nothing new. There is often a putative agent involved. These are very interesting circumstances, but I don't know what more we can say about them."

At the Centers for Disease Control, epidemiologist Matthew Zack, who had not been involved with the original Woburn investigation but who had acquired the unofficial title of "Mr. Cluster" at the Centers by 1984, did not know any more about the study than he had read in the Atlanta papers, but he commented that he was concerned about the methods used and problems of bias. He said, "in cases like this, especially when you rely on a telephone survey, you don't know about the people you did not reach. You don't know if those who did cooperate did so because they had a stake in doing so." And then with characteristic epidemiological two-handedness added, "and you might also say just the reverse. People with illness might be reluctant to talk about it, and that could mean you would miss diseases and introduce bias as well."

Dr. John Cutler, who had been at the heart of the 1980 CDC investigation, said he needed to take a "good look" at the report before making a formal comment but suggested he was somewhat skeptical about the water model used to determine how G and H was distributed. Existence of the model had come as a surprise to him. "When we did our study in 1980," he said with some dismay, "we did not have the water data the DEQE apparently have now. We had a hard time even finding out when those wells went on and off, let alone where the water went."

Some scientists far removed from Woburn appreciated the potential significance immediately of overlaying water distribution patterns with a pattern of disease. Dr. Robert Hoover, who heads the Environmental Studies Section of the National Cancer Institute and who jokes that scientists should talk with their arms tied behind their back "so they can't say 'on the one hand; on the other,'" did comment tentatively: "I can say within my circumscribed knowledge of what actually was done at Woburn, that if you are able to go within a pattern of excess of disease and show it follows the pattern of contaminated drinking water, then that goes a quantum step further toward establishing a credible association."

One prominent cancer epidemiologist with a leading national cancer research institution, who indeed probably should have been provided an advance copy of the Harvard report, had his nose somewhat out of joint because when he telephoned the biostatistics department to request a copy, he was told he would have to pay $10. The department had taken to charging for copies to all but nonprofit organizations. On principle the scientist declined to pay, and as of this writing has yet to read the complete original work.

After the atmosphere of culmination that had prevailed when the Harvard report had been released in Woburn, the initial fairly conservative reception of the report—in particular to what appeared to be the study's unusual features, namely its correlation of birth defects with the well water as well as leukemia—was somewhat puzzling.

Was it simply a question of turf? Zelen and his group were not part of any traditional disease-hunting discipline. They were in private practice, so to speak, in an academic institution, not members of government agencies assigned to protect the public health. They were not hydrology experts or leukemia experts or birth defects experts—they were certainly not traditional epidemiologists. Were they paying a price in credibility for having acted like epidemiologists? Was the institutional skepticism that greeted Anne Anderson and Bruce Young in the first place now being tranferred to the Harvard Department of Biostatistics?

But there was another rather loose end in the subtleties of the results. That the children with leukemia had an average of twice as much of their water coming from wells G and H as other children suggested to Lagakos that the commonality of increased exposure to wells G and H among the leukemic children was very unlikely to be a fluke in itself. Thus he concluded, "because it seems unlikely by chance fluctuation that these children could have had so much exposure while others did not, we concluded that exposure had something to do with their child's being a leukemia case." Plus there seemed to be a "space-time" distribution between the cases and the water, which meant that the leukemia diagnoses came most when and where the wells pumped most water. But still, in the language of statistics, it was hard to pin every single case to very specific exposure to the water. And toward the end of his remarks at Walker Hall, Lagakos said, when asked to express his results in actual numbers of leukemia cases, not in terms of "increased risk," "Of the fifteen leukemia cases diagnosed prior to 1979, three or four could be directly attributable to the wells. The entire increase in cases above what would have been expected could not be statistically explained by the wells." This meant that while all the leukemia children had more exposure, in sum, to G and H water than children without leukemia, not each individual case had higher exposure.

This distinction was not lost on either Anne Anderson or Bruce Young. At lunch shortly after the public meeting they knew that instead of a final answer, they now had a new question before them: Were the Harvard results proof or not?

14

"A Very Blunt Instrument..."

AS SCIENTIFIC QUESTIONS began to swirl around the Harvard study, political pressures were building around the issue of toxic waste in general. In a presidential election year, Ronald Reagan did not wish his administration to become embroiled in a protracted debate about reauthorization of the Superfund legislation. The administration did not push for action, despite the fact that the president had mentioned toxic waste site cleanup as a priority in his 1984 state of the union address.

But Senator Robert Stafford (R-Vermont), who had been a leader in developing the Superfund law in 1980 as chairman of the Senate Environment and Public Works Committee, stated in the spring of 1984, "it is my hope, and I might say, my determination to see a Superfund extension signed into law this year."

To this end, Stafford called hearings on the subject and through the office of Senator Kennedy, several Woburn residents—Anne Anderson, Richard Toomey, Patricia Kane, and Donna Robbins—testified, as well as two other residents of the Silresim site near Lowell. David Ozonoff of Boston University, who had conducted the Silresim study, and Marvin Zelen of Harvard were also called as witnesses.

255

But the volatile issue in the Superfund debate was not the question of extending Superfund monies to local community governments to facilitate the physical clean-up of sites. The trickier business was the question of whether to pass an amendment to the law that would provide compensation to individuals, what became known as the Victims' Compensation Amendment. The amendment had long been opposed by industry and members of Congress, and supporters of the amendment had jettisoned it in the last hours of the 1980 debate as a compromise to allow the Superfund measure itself to pass. But they were trying again in 1984.

In general the concept of victims' compensation would make monies available to individuals who had in some way been harmed personally by release of toxic substances from waste sites. Without such an amendment, individuals had no resort for reimbursement of medical expenses or other costs except to file private toxic tort suits and battle the burden of proof. And in the years since the discovery of the toxic waste problem in Woburn and the contamination of wells G and H, while the Woburn controversy generated funding for scientific studies, high-visibility issues for politicians, dramatic copy for journalists, and potential legal precedents around which attorneys could gravitate, the families of children who were sick or dying had not received a penny to offset the costs they incurred. So the Woburn residents were asked to testify to describe the condition of victims under the Superfund law as it had been passed in 1980.

On April 11, 1984, Anne Anderson and the other witnesses got up at dawn to make their flight. The plane was late, and when they arrived at Washington's National Airport, they were distressed at the idea that they might have missed their slot on the hearing schedule. Yet though they had come to Washington on serious business, they were not solemn. They broke the tension with small talk and jokes about the travail of traveling that surely senators would understand and settled into taxis to take in the brilliance of a warm spring Washington morning. Anne Anderson in particular seemed interested in discerning the rhythm of a busy city already well into the day, chatting with an aide from Senator Kennedy's office about what it would be like to live in the nation's capital.

The hearing room in the Dirksen Office Building was already packed when the Woburn group arrived. All seats in the audience were taken. Two newspaper press tables were full, and behind the arc-shaped dais where nameplates marked the places of senators, half empty, a row of senatorial aides sat against the wall. A battery of television cameras were poised and pointing toward the witness table. Senator Stafford had begun his opening statement, which framed the mission of the hearings in general terms. Then he introduced and paid tribute to the contributions of Senator Randolph, a long-time committee member and supporter of Superfund who would be retiring that year from the Senate after a long career. Then Senator Robert T. Mitchell of Maine also made an introductory statement, reiterating much of what had already been said, and adding the observation that a shortcoming of the previous Superfund legislation was that its provisions could be construed as being applicable to compensate for damage to trees, for example, but not people. The introductory remarks consumed about twenty-five minutes, and the audience was only half listening. Aides came and went from the chamber, and there were still only four senators on the dais reserved for a dozen or so. A camera crew chief snapped his fingers to get the attention of his cameraman and pointed to the people of Woburn.

At about 10 AM, Senator Edward Kennedy entered the hearing room and read a statement urging the passage of the Victims' Compensation Amendment, introducing his constituents, mentioning his own visit to the young Patrick Toomey before his death, and urging his Senate colleagues to "listen well" to the story of Woburn, for the witnesses, he said, "do a real service to this committee and to the country by testifying." He shook hands with each witness before he left the room.

But still more officials had to be heard from, James Florio, congressman from New Jersey, followed by Bill Bradley, senator from New Jersey. Each made a case for versions of the Superfund extension and victims' compensation.

With the end of Bradley's testimony, some senators made jokes about basketball playing, Bradley having been a star basketball player before beginning his Senate career. Senator Randolph then took the opportunity to tell a football joke.

Around this time, Senator Stafford warned the audience that there might be some interruptions ahead because the full Senate was in session and "we are now in danger of a roll call at any minute." The witnesses filed up to the long mahogany witness table. Senator Lautenberg of New Jersey told them their testimony would "be essential to our decision-making processes." Senator Randolph said he hoped he could stay long enough to hear it all, and Senator Stafford, having permitted long greetings and congratulations and poor sports jokes, asked the witnesses to confine their statements to five minutes each.

Anne Anderson began, reading a statement she had written herself, attempting to summarize in the time allowed her the events of the preceding fourteen years of her life.

She gave her name and place of residence and outlined some of the history of her family's move to Woburn. She touched on Jimmy's diagnosis and the evolution of her awareness of other cases, the gradual involvement of Bruce Young, their search to document the number of cases, culminating in the assembly of the amateur cluster map.

As she talked, several senators whispered to their aides who were attempting to conduct other senatorial business during the hearings. Though Anne Anderson had read the statement aloud at home three times to ensure she could make it through without crying, when she spoke of how she had been moved to fight back by seeing her son fight his illness, her voice began to crack.

At the very hint of tears, all present paid attention. Fingers snapped again among the camera crews. All cameras trained on her; the hot lights were brought in closer and glanced back in her face off the mahogany table. Nevertheless she recovered and continued her statement flawlessly:

"We do not think that what has happened in Woburn happened by chance. While we carried our children in our wombs, while we nursed them and weaned them to drink from a cup, we unknowingly offered them the poisons that their bodies could not withstand. . . . We believe our water, water that is so necessary to life itself, was contaminated by the pollutants of industry. I have believed this for a long time, and I have never heard any evidence to convince me I am wrong. Conversely, the more I learn, the more I know, the more convinced I am that our children have suffered and died needlessly. I won't, nor should I be expected to, quietly accept it." No member of the audience spoke a word until she finished.

Pat Kane's testimony related how terrifying a disease like leukemia can be to both parents and children, describing the 176 painful injections Kevin had had to endure in one year, and the extraordinary relief that he had been cured.

Donna Robbins, who had considered asking someone else to read her statement because she was not sure she would find the courage to do so herself, did so with certainty, including a detailed litany of the psychological impact of coping with terminal illness in a child.

She admitted without humiliation that she had been driven to public assistance because of the costs of Robbie's illness but was now graduating from nursing school so she could fend for herself, "for which I can't wait." She ended by simply asking the senators, "what side would you sit on, if you were told that industry contaminated the water you drank, like we drank, if your child was diagnosed with leukemia, like ours were. And just how would you deal with holding your child in your arms as you watched him take his last breath and felt him die?"

The final witness was Richard Toomey, the only man on the panel who was not a scientist and the only father among the families. His first order of business was to tell the senators that it was always difficult for him to relate the facts about Patrick's death and he said, "If I don't make it through, forgive me."

He did, however, describing the incidental expenses that can tend to be overlooked in computing the direct costs of an illness, like parking costs during visits to the hospital, the special treats and toys to reward a child for braving a painful injection, even the cost of replacing the unreliable family car to ensure he would have a vehicle that would get his son to the hospital in time when he needed emergency care. When Richard Toomey finished, he took a long breath and a gulp of water.

Senator Stafford read a prepared statement of thanks to the witnesses and then adjourned the hearings for a recess. Three other committees had been meeting at the same time, and by the end of Richard Toomey's testimony, Stafford was the only senator left in the room.

But when the hearing reconvened, several senators had reappeared. Senator Mitchell of Maine probed more deeply about the magnitude of expenses. The witnesses from Lowell told him they were out of pocket several hundreds to several thousands of dollars for medical care they attributed to their exposure to the site. The Woburn witnesses had more staggering amounts. Anne Anderson said she had never made a complete tally but that in the last year of Jimmy's life, bills for blood transfusions alone were $30,000. Pat Kane added such incidentals as special dentistry costs because Kevin's teeth, like Jimmy Anderson's, had not developed properly because of the leukemia radiation treatments. Donna Robbins estimated that she would have been roughly $200,000 in debt if Robbie's medical expenses had not been covered by public programs. Richard Toomey added up several random piles of bills he had brought with them and got a total of roughly $25,000, which did not include hospitalization costs. While some of the families' medical bills had been reimbursed by medical insurance plans, a bulk had not.

Senator Frank Lautenberg of New Jersey seemed particularly eager to have more epidemiological information. He had become rapt with attention once Anne Anderson began speaking; a press member whispered she had seen Lautenberg wipe away a tear of his own. He had also obviously done some homework during the recess.

Lautenberg told the witnesses "Between this building and the Capitol, where we went to vote, I chanced to meet someone in the Senate who raised the question, 'well how do these people know that the problem, the disease and the sickness to their families, came from their proximity to these sites?' " So, Lautenberg put the question to Woburn families. "How do you know? Is it statistical evidence?" And then feeling out the nub of the issue but still apparently unclear about the extent to which the witnesses had themselves followed the epidemiological studies of Woburn, "Are you aware that the Centers for Disease Control said they found no correlation. . . . I have no doubt that they were wrong. But what does that tell you about the current level of science?"

The hearings had moved into the central question of how a victim could convert the experience of victimization into acceptable proof. Dr. David Ozonoff took a shot at an answer. He characterized the classic epidemiological study, the standard first effort at proof, as "a very blunt instrument with which to dissect very delicate personal tragedies."

Continuing in a metaphorical mode, he compared epidemiologists attempting to use conventional assessment methods to gauge effects of toxic waste exposure to "people who go into a huge dark warehouse full of dangerous objects wearing a miner's lamp. They don't see anything and walk out again and say there was nothing there. . . . Their power to see things is too small."

Ozonoff described his Silresim study and argued that because of the limitations of science, and just plain lack of people power, the chances of missing effects that occur approximately once in every 200 people were quite high. "The best way," he added, "to find no relationship is to do an inadequate study."

Then Marvin Zelen testified about the biostatistics department analysis of the effects of wells G and H. He admitted that such studies, "by their nature," cannot prove cause and effect, but he added, "the aggregate of evidence was overwhelming that the availability of water from those two wells is positively associated with adverse health affects." He also added some new information that had not been announced publicly in Woburn. He was convinced of his further analysis of the birth defect data and was sure that the rates of birth defects had evened out after the closing of wells G and H in 1979. Of the leukemia rate, he said, "it is still high, and that could continue for awhile, but there have been no new cases of leukemia in the areas that received most of the well water." Zelen said he hoped that from the Woburn study, some "national strategy" for assessing health patterns at toxic waste sites would emerge.

When the hearings adjourned, the Woburn group relaxed, and some hugged each other.

They knew intuitively that it had only been their suffering that had thrust them onto center stage, and they projected both relief that the testimony was over and the hope that maybe it would bring about legislative changes that would help others like themselves.

They spent the afternoon talking with the congressional staff, just missed the last direct flight home, and so did not reach Woburn again before 11 PM or so. It had been a long and draining day, but they felt it had been worthwhile. As Anne Anderson said, "we were all exhausted, but we felt satisfied because we had done an important thing that no one else could have done."

As it turned out, they had, and they hadn't, for even the basic Superfund extension legislation did not pass that year. Though Democratic presidential nominee Walter Mondale used a shot of himself visiting Woburn in his nominating convention film, and Congresswoman Geraldine Ferraro took a break from her vice-presidential campaign to argue on the floor of the House for a Superfund extension, most sitting politicians knew it was unlikely that such potentially volatile political issues would be put to a final congressional vote on the eve of a presidential election.

One wonders if it had been truly realistic for Superfund proponents to expect to win more money for Superfund at a time when the only election issue that seemed able to hold public attention was the extent of the national debt. Probably the testimony of the Woburn families would have been ultimately more effective had it been heard by a fully attentive, fully participating committee not distracted by the short-lived dialogues of a presidential campaign.

While the issue of victims' compensation had come in and out of legislative focus in the larger Superfund discussions throughout the election year, the Harvard biostatistics department study itself also attracted attention.

In fact, just two weeks or so after the Stafford hearings, a memo had reached the desk of the then head of the EPA, William Ruckelshaus, from the assistant EPA administrator for research and development, headed simply "re: Woburn." However, the memo referred specifically and only to an ongoing review by the department's office of research and development of the Zelen study, referred to as the "Harvard Study reporting adverse health consequences in relationship to water contamination in Woburn."

The ongoing review had apparently begun shortly after the public release of the Zelen study.

It is a curious memo, even allowing for the fact that it was a preliminary document based on preliminary interpretations of the Harvard results. The memo had a question-and-answer format and opens with the least important aspect of what was contained in the Harvard study, namely what the researchers had known when they started, that there had been a cluster of leukemia. The EPA memo says, "the [Harvard] evidence strongly suggests that there is an unexpectedly high incidence of childhood leukemia in Woburn which has been present since at least the late 1960s." Then, however, the memo says "perhaps the most convincing finding in this regard is the fact that there has been a persistent increase in leukemia incidence since the original cluster of cases was evaluated in 1979."

For one thing, the original cluster was not evaluated until 1981. It was the wells that were closed in 1979. And the cases characterized as representing a "persistent increase" were in fact the four cases to which Lagakos had himself called attention at the public meeting. But whereas Lagakos had said that they indeed represented a lingeringly high rate, he had also said that given the latency period for leukemia, a high rate could be expected to continue for awhile after the wells were shut down. Lagakos had also noted that the "new" cases were conceived before the wells were shut down, making them "new" in the sense of diagnosis date only. Use of the words "persistent increase since 1979" in the EPA memo gave the impression the leukemia rate was actually climbing since the wells were closed, not trailing off.

The second paragraph, which was meant to answer the question "is childhood leukemia in Woburn associated with exposure to contaminated groundwater?" further garbled the Harvard research strategy and the essence of its results: "The evidence for such an association [between leukemia and groundwater] is much less than compelling. If one looks at the cases reported up until 1979, there is some suggestive but weak evidence of an association with drinking water from two contaminated wells. The data do not follow the expected dose–latency period relationship. It must be emphasized that these wells were closed in 1979. Only one of the four new cases of childhood leukemia had any exposure to the two contaminated wells, and this was minimal. Inasmuch as these four new cases are the linchpin for confirming that a real problem exists in Woburn, ascribing this problem to groundwater contamination is highly questionable."

But the four new cases, far from being the "linchpin" for confirming there was a problem, were, if anything, suggestive that the problem might not be the wells at all.

In its concluding paragraph the memo essentially dismisses the Harvard data on birth defects.

In short, although the memo made it all the way to the desk of the nation's leading environmental protection officer, it almost completely misinterpreted the results of the study and seemed to entirely miss the point of its strategy. It made no reference to the larger goal the study hoped to achieve: an enhancement of conventional epidemiological methods for evaluating health effects of toxic waste sites. Whereas one might have expected such a study to capture attention for what could be learned from it, the EPA ongoing review seemed to focus solely, and erroneously, on what the report failed to prove.

The memo was described a year after it was written as the agency's "initial scientific opinion," which had not benefited from an examination of the data "underlying the Harvard report," namely, the water model. But not seeing the water model could not explain the errors in the memo, or more importantly, its tone.

The memo effectively minimized the Harvard find-

ings, and though it suggested that the EPA was interested enough in the Harvard study to review it very
quickly, it did not convey a constructive let's-roll-
up-our-sleeves-and-see-what-can-be-learned-from-this
approach. In fact, EPA's "ongoing review" of the study
consisted of not a single direct conversation with Marvin
Zelen and only one brief conversation with Steven
Lagakos.

The negative interpretation of the Harvard report
found other outlets. Dr. Renate Kimbrough, a well-
known epidemiologist and long-time associate at the
CDC, presented her review of the Harvard-Woburn
Health study in May 1984 at a hearing held by the Massachusetts State Legislature on the possibilities of implementing a state-based victims' compensation plan.

She had studied the health effects of dioxin exposures
and had investigated such substances as pentochloro-
phenol, a wood preservative, and its effects on the health
of people who live in prefabricated log cabins presumably doused with the substance. The chemical was
banned for use in the United States in 1984.

Dr. Kimbrough focused her remarks on the methods
Zelen and Lagakos used and what she perceived as a
lack of explanation for them in the copy of the study she
had. She wondered about how the town of Woburn had
been divided for the purposes of the survey and how it
was decided which FACE volunteers would call which
numbers, and she objected to some of the disease groupings—such as Down's syndrome appearing in a group
along with spina bifida—since these diseases have "different etiologies" or different known causes. Kimbrough's objection was based on the clinical nature of

the cases. Indeed they present very different symptoms and different gross biological causes. But their underlying causes, a genetic abnormality, is precisely the sort of abnormality with which toxic contamination is associated. In other words, although the Harvard group acknowledged their disease groupings were clinically imperfect, they claimed that they consciously grouped the diseases because they might have a common underlying cause, if not a common immediate cause. It was the difference in approaches between a statistician and a physician.

There is a hint between the lines in the criticism that the Harvard group was attempting to "put something over." For example, Dr. Kimbrough says, "The questions in the questionnaire are rather open-ended, and although the authors of the report state that they adjusted for smoking in their analyses, there are no such questions [about smoking] listed on the questionnaire." In fact, smoking habit data is requested in question 5.

Dr. Kimbrough also took on the model of water distribution in Woburn, correctly pointing out that it had not been independently verified. But she referred to original CDC information about water distribution as if what had been known about Woburn water distribution in 1980 had been more sophisticated than the information Harvard used. In fact, what the CDC had used in 1980 came from basic town records and was nowhere near as complex as what the DEQE provided Harvard.

Throughout her criticism, Dr. Kimbrough, of the CDC, referred to the CDC report as if it were a touchstone to which the Harvard study should be compared, and not the other way around.

Yet, after saying several times in her remarks that she was "not impressed" that the contamination of wells G and H had any effect on disease in Woburn, she concludes, "From the latest Woburn study, I am not able to draw any conclusions as to whether any of the reported health problems are associated with living in Woburn." Dr. Kimbrough acknowledges she did not have time to review the appendix of the Harvard report, which contained much of the underlying explanation for their statistical methods and their disease groupings.

Dr. Kimbrough was joined in her criticism of the biostatistics study at the same hearings by Dr. Brian MacMahon, an especially significant development, since he is a noted epidemiologist based essentially down the hall from Zelen and his team, namely as chairman of the Epidemiology Department at the Harvard School of Public Health.

MacMahon sternly laced into the Zelen report, criticizing the "medical naivete of grouping diverse birth defects such as nervous system abnormalities and chromosomal abnormalities" under the broad heading "environmentally associated disease." He also criticized the study for failing to reach 47% of the target population.

The public criticism of a close colleague was rather unorthodox and eventually made its way to the *Boston Globe* on June 8 under a page 21 headline, "Authors' Colleague Raps Woburn Study." MacMahon was quoted as having told the *Globe*, "I think it is a very bad study. . . poorly planned. It ignored many precepts of epidemiology or community surveys that we have known about for a long time, and I think it was much over interpreted."

MacMahon admitted he had been asked by the American Industrial Health Council to serve on an industry-sponsored review of the Harvard biostatistics report, had accepted, but then declined. He also declined to be interviewed for this book, even about general questions in epidemiology, on the grounds that he did not wish to be in the position of "criticizing a colleague in public."

For their parts, Zelen and Lagakos were described as "flabbergasted" by MacMahon's comments. While they obviously had not asked MacMahon for advice on the study design, they did tell the *Globe* he had declined to discuss his objections to it when they invited him to do so. Marvin Zelen, reached on his sabbatical, refused to answer MacMahon's charges because he had not heard MacMahon's statements personally, except to say, "If Dr. MacMahon is being quoted correctly, it looks to me as if his comments are quite superficial and don't indicate that he has read the study carefully."

The feud broke wide open and moved to yet another forum, a seminar held at the Harvard School of Public Health, where Dr. MacMahon expanded and repeated his criticism. Transcripts of his remarks were made available to the press by the W. R. Grace Company. And in that bad feelings between scientists seemed both between and squarely on the lines, the seminar hardly set new standards for professional discourse.

On June 22, 1984, Lagakos opened the seminar with a review of the study findings and its methods. He was followed by Dr. MacMahon who said, "Three items of introduction. First, for those already weary, let me tell you that this is not going to be your usual ten-minute discussion. I plan in fact to speak for about thirty minutes. Since I am not normally so long-winded, I must explain that I was, in effect, challenged—it is not too strong a word—by Dr. Zelen and Dr. Lagakos to repeat, in public, remarks I made to the Massachusetts Commission on Liability for Release of Hazardous Materials. Having taken up the gauntlet I cannot flippantly dispose of the matter in ten minutes.

"Second, I want to thank Dr. Lagakos for taking the time to explain to me a number of points that none of the manuscripts made clear to my unmathematical mind.

"Third, I must express my discomfort at discussing so formally a series of manuscripts of which the final version is not yet in the public domain . . . partly I face a moving target. Should I discuss the twenty-one page "synopsis" that was released when the findings were first announced on February 8; the blue-covered report which appeared at the same time but was either rapidly withdrawn or outstocked; the second edition of the blue-covered report distinguished by the outline of Woburn on the cover; the manuscript submitted for scientific publication, or the presentation we have heard here today?"

The MacMahon remarks continued in the same vein. "It is my purpose," MacMahon told his audience, "to persuade you of my view that the Woburn study is much less than the definitive demonstration of the ill-health effects of careless chemical waste disposal that the newspapers and regulators are regarding it to be."

The part of the study pertaining to the actual leukemia cluster, MacMahon said, "disturbs me least." He wondered how the cases had been verified and wished—

"it would have been nice"—to know what cell type the leukemias were. The cell types of the cluster, of course, had already been verified by the CDC in 1981. Mac-Mahon expanded his criticism of the groupings of the other types of diseases by calling the categories "meaningless" and said he was not persuaded that the association between the wells and the leukemia cases was "geographic" with respect to individual households. Of course, no one had ever said the water model was as specific as how much water went into each individual house; the model simply provided a look at the distribution by region, down to the level of a group of streets. But the model was certainly more refined than a gross distinguishing of East Woburn from West, which is what Dr. MacMahon implied.

MacMahon thought the use of volunteers practically voided the validity of any of the study results. He concluded that it was impossible to regard any of the findings with "any degree of confidence."

Then he tossed out the most subjective ball of all. He asked "is there anything to be learned from the Woburn study? I think there is. The study was conceived in politics. That is not an accusation—almost any study in an applied field shares this characteristic. But in this instance the politics dictated not only that a study should be done but the time frame within which it should be completed, which in turn put constraints on the resources which were available to the investigators and imposed even other constraints on the design features of the enquiry. Here we have a recipe for failure that not even the remarkable statistical talents of this eminent group of investigators was able to avert."

MacMahon was right that the Harvard report had gone through a number of editorial permutations since its public release in Woburn in February, but the final results had been substantially the same. Also public release, prior to release in a scientific peer review journal, had been unorthodox and was perhaps needlessly provocative. And to be sure, the biostatistics department did gain some laurels by appearing to be the only scientific body truly responsive to the community's concerns. However, what of this "politics"?

Did MacMahon mean to imply that his colleagues were no more than hired henchmen of the inflamed Woburn community and that they were pressed to do a study that "found something"? Would Harvard and the Dana Farber Cancer Institute have underwritten such a project to the tune of half a million dollars of service donated in kind?

Or was it simply that Zelen and Lagakos, widely regarded as outstanding biostatisticians, were themselves so personally motivated to "get" toxic waste dumpers that they were willing to do a sloppy study, leaving them open to professional criticism from virtually every quarter?

And what of this "time frame"? Did Dr. MacMahon mean that Dr. Zelen wanted to get away on his sabbatical, or was he subtly suggesting that the study had to come out quickly so that it could be used in private litigation as well as public discussion on the matter of victims' compensation? If so, who asked Zelen and Lagakos to rush? Was it FACE? Was it Bruce Young and Anne Anderson? Was it enemies of industry in the Massachusetts Legislature or the United States Congress?

It would seem that the "politics" and the "time frame" applied more to the criticism of the study than the inception of the study. Within a few weeks of its release the report was being scrutinized in the office of the head of the EPA, who was being provided incorrect basic information, and it was being villified by epidemiologists in front of a state commission largely for not speaking the language of epidemiology. An industrial health council was convened to review the material, but the reviewers made no arrangement to talk directly with Zelen or Lagakos.

In short, instead of examining the Harvard study— despite its imperfections, most of which Zelen and Lagakos had themselves anticipated at the outset and attempted to correct—for its creative approach to a problem that seemed locked in a rut, some of the most noted epidemiologists in the country plunged into the business of tearing it apart. Not one of them, however, offered to do a better study that might enhance the body of knowledge.

Just as in the days of Snow and Virchow and Kelsch, disbelief came more easily than faith, and scientific rivalry, personality conflicts, and institutional jealousies did not die just because some children did.

The fact is that no epidemiological study is perfect. Perfection eludes each and every one of them. The nature of the epidemiological approach is limited in many ways these scientists readily admit. So why hang Harvard for its brand of imperfections? Why not instead take that roll-up-the-sleeves cooperative attitude and attempt to build on what Harvard had begun?

Perhaps because of the rut in which traditional epidemiology by definition finds itself in relationship to environmental hazards, and because biostatistics and hydrogeologists and concerned parents cannot as easily be regarded as allies as they can be perceived as interlopers?

And perhaps because if the community of Woburn could find proof, then there might be ramifications for all the towns around America with toxically contaminated water and those who caused the contamination.

The report by the American Industrial Health Council on the Harvard Biostatistics Study, released in October 1984, largely expanded and echoed the previous criticism. It raised some new items: that the entire study was based on the assumption that only wells G and H were contaminated and not others in the city and that the study failed to properly control for socioeconomic status of the respondents, which might have tended to account for where the respondents were living.

There had indeed been evidence that G and H wells were the only contaminated water sources in Woburn. And East Woburn is a middle-class community with little real sociological variation block to block. While there are certainly life-style factors that can influence the development of cancer, such as diet, it would be hard to accept that life-style factors could have accounted for the original leukemia cluster.

Clearly no one is served by the conduct of sloppy science. But given the truly complex nature of understanding the role of ambient environmental contamination in health patterns, one wonders what kind of study could possibly please everybody?

It can be instructive to look at a study designed by

one of the leading detractors of the Harvard study. Dr. Patricia Buffler of the University of Texas is herself a well-known epidemiologist and served on the American Industrial Health Council review panel for the Harvard report. In a long telephone interview, she said of the Zelen team, "I was appalled by their naivete and the approach."

At the time she reviewed the Harvard report, she was deeply immersed in her own epidemiological work following up what appeared to be increased incidences of various types of brain cancers among employees in the petrochemical industries of the coastal areas of Texas. There is no question that the study had been fastidiously designed and was large in scope. It sought to evaluate six Texas counties and twenty-six Louisiana parishes, surveying a population of 3.5 million people in Texas and 2 million in Louisiana. All newly diagnosed cases confirmed by a pathologist's review of the tumorous tissue would be included. Diagnoses were further corroborated by a detailed review of hospital medical records. In fact, a special two-day training session for medical record keepers was held by the study team to make sure diagnoses were standardized and that the types of tumors being studied were in fact the same type.

Because of the large general population the study was sampling, it expected to find some 300 cases of the tumors in Texas, plus 200 in Louisiana, and these approximately 500 cases would be matched with identical control subjects. Once the medical records were reviewed and it was established that each case was in fact a case, the patient or next of kin would be interviewed in order to see if there were common factors of residential pattern, workplace exposures, diets, hobbies, and medical treatments. If a residential pattern were to be discovered, the study group might recommend several million dollars of air and water monitoring of the residential areas to see if there were contaminants present associated with brain cancer.

The study was also being designed to determine whether advanced techniques for detecting brain cancers could account for the increased incidence by having made it easier to actually identify the type of tumor being investigated, thus contributing to higher numbers of cases overall.

Data would be collected through the fall of 1985 and analyzed after that. Interviewers were intensively trained, and the interviewer manual of directions was nearly 2 inches thick. All patients and controls were to be quizzed about other illnesses from which they might suffer, and detailed medical, residential, and employment histories were to be taken.

The study would not actually measure workplace exposures, except by job category. It would depend on the patient or next of kin to report on job history. In other words, interviewers would not actually go into petrochemical plants and measure what chemicals were present. Neither would they measure chemical exposures inside individual homes. And the study did not plan to recommend environmental sampling of air and water unless it found a residential pattern of illness.

Dr. Buffler concedes the problem of quantifying environmental exposures connected to specific jobs without having taken physical measurements in the workplace, and of measuring ambient pollutants in neighborhoods many years after the fact. But the study, she said, was carefully controlled against any other sort of bias.

In other words, though the study is an absolutely meticulously planned piece of epidemiological work, obviously cautious to eliminate great and small potential biases, it was virtually predestined to come to a stone wall.

It would not be able to go further than to say that a pattern of brain cancer was or was not associated with a pattern of residence; it would not be able to say more than a pattern of brain cancer was or was not associated with a particular job description.

It would not be able to name or quantify specific substances because no physical measurements would be taken in workplaces. If it takes physical measurements in residential areas, it will do so many years after the latency factor for the cancers in question, and most clues are likely to be gone.

In other words, the study will be inherently unable to come closer to understanding any specific relationships between the petrochemical industry and brain cancer than was possible before the study was undertaken. It is the sort of beautiful research that cannot help pin cause to effect.

15

The Case of the "New" Cases

IN MARCH 1985 the United States Office of Technology Assessment released a report which said that instead of there being 2,500 "priority toxic waste sites" in the United States, as previously estimated by the EPA, there were likely to be more than 10,000 in the priority category. Instead of costs for cleanup reaching approximately $20 billion, as estimated by the EPA, the costs could approach $100 billion. And overall that instead of there being approximately 25,000 priority and lesser priority waste sites, the number of sites definable as "hazardous," on the basis of the nature of the substances they contain and the cleanup action they require, could climb ultimately as high as 378,000.

The report also cited the relatively slow progress on cleanup of waste sites, noting that of the 538 sites identified by the EPA at that point as deserving of priority attention, only thirty were in some stage of remediation.

For Woburn's 300-acre Industri-Plex Superfund site, this meant that as of spring 1985 not a single drop of liquid contamination or a shovelful of contaminated soil had been removed from the site. In fact, in the spring of 1985, Woburn firemen were called upon to extinguish a fire in a field near the arsenic pits at Industri-Plex and

280

were subsequently hospitalized for tests to determine if they had absorbed ambient arsenic into their blood. Except for the Cyclone fencing and barbed wire strung around the site personally by Robert Cleary and Richard Leighton back in the early 1980s, and a handful of "danger" signs, the site remained virtually exactly as it was when it was discovered in 1979.

In fact, even after the site was defined by the fence, toxic waste was still being discovered in parts of Woburn. In West Woburn, several miles away from Industri-Plex, for example, in 1984, a family was having its backyard excavated with the intention of putting in a swimming pool, and as workers dug down deeper, it was as though they had hit a Minoan road. A large concrete slab appeared as dirt was pushed aside, which ultimately proved to be a concrete vault filled with toxic sludge apparently abandoned by a defunct and long-since-razed animal degreasing plant that had taken up the equivalent of a city block. The chamber contained chromium sludge, as well as naphtha, a substance commonly used to take oil out of animal hides. The soil above the chamber also contained naphtha. Five homes sat on the tract of land. No further excavations were done at the time to determine whether more chambers existed. The brook that runs behind the property, which feeds the Horn Pond aquifer, an important source of drinking water in Woburn, was found to be free of naphtha, however.

As the professional criticism of the Harvard study subsided, and there were few new developments in Woburn, the issue of relationship of the wells to the leukemia cluster moved to the institutional back burner.

Yet through the summer of 1984, FACE continued to function, with Anne Anderson and Bruce Young perfecting their records of the leukemia cases. They also gave testimony at various commissions at work on public health issues. Other members of the organization worked with local teachers to develop science class curriculums for students on the issues of toxic waste. FACE also kept tabs on water quality at Horn Pond, pointing out that in periods of heavy rains, sewer and street runoff headed for the pond and compromised its quality. The DEQE continued to investigate sources of contamination of the groundwater feeding wells G and H, but otherwise things in Woburn were quiet. Then came what might be called the case of the "new" cases.

In November of 1984 the Massachusetts Department of Public Health (MDPH) released results of an "update" it had completed in August that year of childhood leukemia in Woburn. The department announced that the rate of childhood leukemia had continued to be elevated and that it had found seven "new" cases of leukemia diagnosed since 1980, that is, after wells G and H were closed. The commissioner of health, Bailus Walker, told the press his department had "continued to monitor" the leukemia incidence in Woburn since its January 1981 report and that, assuming the wells had been implicated, "we had hoped to see a decrease in the number of new childhood cases in Woburn, but unfortunately this has not happened." Walker continued, "In light of our recent update, we believe that an independent expert review of available information on the relationship between environmental contamination and child health in Woburn will help us identify additional avenues of inquiry." Walker announced that such an expert panel was being convened with a grant from the Centers for Disease Control (CDC).

But the "new" cases were not in fact as new as all that. For one thing, it is clear from the memorandum generated by Commissioner Walker's office that the department's "update" in fact consisted mainly of a review of a list "furnished by the Rev. Bruce Young," a list in fact compiled by Anderson and Young, plus three additional cases reported as having been treated at the Dana-Farber Cancer Institute in Boston. In fact, despite the official nature of the update, it was obvious that Bruce Young and Anne Anderson were still the best available sources for comprehensive information on the number of leukemia cases.

Perhaps more to the point, the new cases were not new to all. Four of the seven were the very four that Lagakos had mentioned at the Woburn public meeting back in February 1984, acknowledging that this number represented a continued elevated rate but that given leukemia latency, it was too soon to expect to see a decline. Doubtlessly these four cases were also the same four characterized in the April 23 memo to William Ruckelshaus as a "persistent increase." But the effect of calling the cases new was to suggest that exposure to wells G and H had not been involved.

However, several significant points got lost in the newness shuffle. Only one of the seven new cases was found in the East Woburn areas where most of the G and H water was distributed, which might suggest that the wells did not account for new cases after they were closed. This would tend to confirm their possible causal role in leukemias that appeared before the wells ceased operation. And only two of the children diagnosed since 1980 were conceived after the wells were shut down, a pattern also consistent with involvement of the wells in the original leukemia cluster. Also, in discussing the newness of the cases the MDPH made no mention of the latency factor. At other times in discussing Woburn the MDPH had used two to five years as the generally accepted latent period for childhood leukemia, and that is indeed when the incidence of the disease among children peaks. But, according to a review of the clustering phenomenon published in the book *Cancer Epidemiology and Prevention*, latency has a "well-defined maximum, which is the time from the child's conception to his disease onset." If this definition is used, the wells could have caused leukemia in any child conceived prior to their shutdown and who was exposed to the well water, regardless of the diagnosis date.

In short, instead of diminishing the significance of the role of the wells—thereby diminishing the significance of the Harvard findings—the "new" cases actually suggested new, intriguing considerations. First, that the leukemia incidence rate had not declined could simply mean that Woburn had two—not one—clusters, a "pre–well closing" and a "post–well closing" cluster. A post-1979 cluster in terms of diagnosis might still contain cases in which the wells may have played a part. Too, the diagnoses since 1980, which seem unrelated to the wells, might indeed be flukes of chance, but this need not negate the fact that the pre-1980 diagnoses may have been brought on by well exposure.

Finally the increased incidence of leukemia outside

what was generally regarded as the area where well G and H water distributed on the basis of the draft DEQE water model could mean that the model was not entirely correct and that at times well G and H water may have reached areas other than just East Woburn. Certainly in 1978 when well G was pumping nonstop, it is possible that its water reached homes beyond the original tight East Woburn leukemia circle. And too, contaminated residue could have lingered in the plumbing system after the wells were closed.

Summarizing all the uncertainties raised by the "new" case scenario, John Cutler, who had been at first skeptical of the role of the wells, said simply, "it is too early to say what the role of the wells actually was one way or the other."

But the new cases announcement did enable the MDPH to take the lead, and it meant an expert panel, under the auspices of the CDC, could be called in at the request of the state health department. Thus, continuing investigation in Woburn would not be perceived as a "catch-up" strategy, or a response to the Harvard study and the attention it received. After all, in theory the MDPH or the CDC could have stayed on the matter of how well G and H water distributed in Woburn after 1981, and when the DEQE model became available, either of those agencies could have commissioned its own biostatistical study, rather than wait to see an independent university department develop the idea.

Although the concept of an expert review panel was publicly attributed to the agency's concern that the leukemia incidence had not declined as "hoped," the panel was likely a result of the impetus and national stature given the Woburn events by the Harvard study and the study's provocative nature. But, coming hard on the heels of the news conference announcing the "update-new cases" scenario, the summoning of an expert panel looked like a public agency initiative and not a reaction to a ripple set in motion by a private academic institution.

Also the MDPH had made much of the fact that the Woburn cluster was different from virtually all others because, unlike other clusters investigated by the CDC where the disease clumping and higher incidence had disappeared as mysteriously as it began, the high Woburn rate persisted. This lingering effect, the department said, suggested the need for continuing department concern and involvement. But, first, one must wonder if indeed all other leukemia clusters have simply "disappeared." Certainly not every cluster investigation has been as continuously and closely monitored as Woburn, and it is doubtful that there is any authoritative source for saying all previous leukemia clusters—which are only the clusters that have come to light—have disappeared. It may be true, but it cannot be authoritatively known. It is not even authoritatively known how many leukemia clusters there have been. It is only known how many cancer clusters overall the CDC investigated on an initial basis, which is 101 since 1963. Of these, very few, according to Dr. Glyn Caldwell, were followed up, and the basis for saying clusters usually disappeared, according to Caldwell, was actually that "we [the CDC] ceased hearing about them or having people ask us to look into them." The CDC never kept up with Rutherford, New Jersey, for example. Nor did it follow up Unicoi County, Tennessee, to know whether that cluster in fact disappeared. Usually once the CDC has done an initial epidemiological verification that the cluster exists, follow-up is left to the state health departments.

So the statement that clusters usually disappear can in part be a function of nobody knowing otherwise.

Though the "update" announcement on one hand gave the impression that the MDPH wished to stay on top of a dynamic situation, on the other, the implicit message was that if there had been no "new" cases, wells G and H would have been more definitely implicated, and the department would have been more likely to have left it at that.

Which is, in fact, exactly what had happened in January 1981 and where Woburn matters would have ended had FACE given up and the Harvard study not come along to toss another pebble into the pool.

And while publicly, for example, few public health officials would embrace the Harvard results while they were being so hotly criticized, privately, John Cutler mentioned, "most people are satisfied that the Harvard study explained those early leukemia cases," meaning the cases pre-1979, and he added that the bickering at Harvard should be "taken with a grain of salt."

The pronounced movement of the MDPH around the "new cases" did tend to look like the institution wanted to capture the outfront position. Indeed a February 1984 report on the environmental health needs of the state of Massachusetts submitted to the commissioner of public health in February 1984 had been critical of the department. The report, prepared by a study group convened by the incoming commissioner in 1983, had suggested that the department suffered from lack of management skills among some senior personnel; there was a tendency to put out fires rather than to develop an overall plan. Also, the department did not enjoy high credibility among the public at large or local health officials who thought that the department frequently failed to follow through on initial actions that it took. A large part of the impetus for establishing the study group had been generated by the Woburn events.

But no institution is faceless, and every person at work in any large organization has individual career goals, insecurities, personal motives, a need to be recognized, a need to be right, and above all a need to avoid being shown to be wrong. These are human motivations, often operating unconsciously. As the baton of public attention passed from one Woburn development to the next in the early 1980s, the institutions responsible responded through the individuals at hand.

And when the Woburn events first erupted and Anderson and Young were clamoring for someone to pay attention to their findings, the state's environmental response mechanism consisted of three persons responsible for meeting the needs of 621 cities and towns. This miserable allocation of human resources reflected, of course, a miserly allocation of financial resources. To increase one's allocation requires a battle to justify one's program. The corollary of this technique is the "dejustification" of programs, recognized as the best strategy for cutting away budget funds, say observers of David Stockman and his federal budget-cutting process under the Reagan administration.

So it could be said that the "new cases" announcement was partly to "justify" the approximately $34,000 appropriation made to the MDPH by the CDC through the Superfund program by citing a need to go into action. The department could not say to the CDC, "we need this money to follow leads uncovered by Bruce Young and Anne Anderson years ago," but that is what the money and the panel implicitly meant.

In fact, if progress in a situation like Woburn's can be measured by the amount of study they receive, the expert panel convened at Woburn did represent a bold, unprecedented, and creative move. No previous cluster investigation had ever gotten this far before in that the panel, composed of experts from various disciplines— hydrology, statistics, genetics, pediatrics, epidemiology, even sociology—had been called together to collectively eyeball a particular environmental problem. And a panel of mixed and erudite composition did not seem like a panel put together to reinvent the wheel. Indeed, where the previous cluster investigations had been hampered by the limits of the traditional epidemiological method, finding commonality but having to stop at causality, the mixing of expertises held the promise that new angles and new ingredients could be introduced.

The MDPH held a preliminary planning hearing in Woburn in January 1985, a process conceived by Elaine Krueger, chief of the Environmental Toxicology Unit of the MDPH, specifically to solicit input from the community. About thirty people came to the hearing, which was held at city hall with the mayor in attendance. Ms. Krueger said that the panel would be looking for creative ways to investigate the cluster mystery. Mayor Rabbitt then presented her with a piece of iron water pipe, fairly whistle clean, that Anne Anderson had suggested be cut from the Montvale Road section of East Woburn. The pipe, the mayor told Kreuger, had been in place a long time, and yet it was almost free of rust and sediment. Was it perhaps that years of solvent water contamination could have left the pipe so clean? It was not a far-fetched idea, and Kreuger did bring the pipe to the panel's attention. As it turned out, chlorine use might have been responsible for some of the cleanliness of the pipe, but probably not all.

Then the experts themselves came to Woburn to hear community sentiment. In February of 1985 approximately 100 people attended, this time at the Woburn High School, a far cry from the days before FACE had its Main Street office, when Bruce Young was told by town officials that FACE was an unofficial organization and therefore could not use official buildings, like schools, to hold public meetings.

The expert panel received copies of the 1981 CDC and MDPH reports on Woburn, a small map of the cluster cases, and two press clips. They interviewed principals in the further research, like Marvin Zelen, and they were taken on a bus tour of Woburn, each presumably viewing the front yards and ranch houses and tannery smoke stacks and abandoned well stations from their own unique professional perspective. Then they began to ruminate and make recommendations.

In June 1985 the panel's report was made public, and it represented probably the most comprehensive set of suggestions for finding answers ever made by the scientific community about Woburn. Its suggestions for further study and monitoring indeed notched the Woburn investigation onto a level where, maybe, something could be learned from it. The panel's reasoning was fourfold.

It first reaffirmed concern about the "new" cases.

Its second reason rekindled an old story, thanks no doubt to the presence of a virologist on the panel, the first virologist who had ever spoken with the Woburn community about its leukemia problems, the first virologist to look in detail at the Woburn cluster, for that matter. The panel said, "scientific advances have clarified the role of viruses and genetic processes in rare forms of childhood cancer in humans and in animals. One might, for instance, speculate that a viral agent 'caused' some of the previously reported clusters in children, but that new techniques were not available to discover it. The opportunity for a sophisticated search for cause should not be lost."

Third, the panel considered the wells and their relationship to both old and new cases and said, "a putative cause, exposure to contaminated water, has been proposed and investigated in this community. While the strength of the supporting evidence is debatable, there is no basis for ruling out this possibility at the present time."

A fourth reason for urging further study was the "evidence of the unusually pervasive presence of multiple environmental toxins" in the Woburn community.

The panel took pains to note that it wanted to respond directly to a "theme raised several times in community meetings, for Woburn to be regarded as a model or exemplary community in terms of public health watchfulness for adverse health effects." In other words, if there was an environmental villain afoot in Woburn, the panel acknowledged that the only way to find it was to go out and look intensively for it.

First the panel recommended an exhaustive complete list of all leukemia cases be made—perhaps not realizing that the resources of FACE would be essential here since Anne Anderson and Bruce Young were accustomed to keeping such lists. The panel recommended the list be monitored closely for the next few years; it recommended that virtually every stream and well in Woburn be checked for chemical contamination, along with extensive indoor and outdoor sampling of air and a routine screen test for lead exposure in the blood of Woburn children, as part of their routine pediatric care; it suggested that "encouragement should be given to researchers to characterize fully in the laboratory the cell type and chromosomal aberrations present in existing and incident cases of childhood leukemia in Woburn"; the suggestion was made that blood and tissue samples be taken of any child diagnosed with leukemia as the diagnosis came in, preferably before chemotherapy begins, the idea being that even if these specimens told no tale now, in the future researchers might be able to learn something from them as techniques and knowledge develop.

The panel also recommended a full-scale health monitoring program, including laboratory tests to search out genetic damage, to study rates of defects in children—like cardiac anomalies and limb and facial defects—as well as fetal deaths. And on top of all this the panel recommended a public education program for the community and practical coordination between all agencies involved, namely the CDC, the MDPH, EPA, and the DEQE.

It was, finally, an enormous plan for watching health in Woburn, indeed the blueprint for a living laboratory. The panel made no reference to cost, but certainly its price tag will be in the millions, and it is doubtful all the monies required can be easily found. And though the panel's recommendations are indeed probably the only way to learn what has been going on in Woburn, it is hard to know how such a program could meet one of the panel's own internal criteria—namely, that its recommendations be "undisturbing" to the community once implemented. But if Woburn had been concerned about image and real estate values when Edward Kennedy toured Industri-Plex in a special "moon suit" to protect him from toxic vapors, what would happen when prospective newcomers to town are told the price of admission includes lead and chromosomal screening tests for adults and children?

Welcome to Woburn and thousands of other communities in the United States where toxic waste has been recognized to be a potential health problem!

What is clear from the panel's report is that an effective program of health monitoring from which something could truly be learned cannot help but be both expensive and intrusive. The alternative is to learn nothing at all.

Of course, there are several implicit messages in the panel report. For one thing, though the panel concluded, "the possibility cannot be discounted that the Woburn cluster will disappear in the same way as have the others," one wonders if such a panel would recommend a multi-million dollar program simply to extinguish the theory that the clustering had not happened by chance alone. So one can extrapolate that the panel was at least moderately persuaded that something had happened in Woburn to cause the cluster and that something could be found.

The emphasis on viruses is fascinating and ironic. It not only leads back to the 1950s and early theories about cancer causation, but also to an original instinct of Anne Anderson, who had been reading about leukemia viruses in connection with learning about Jimmy's disease, that the smelly water could be carrying a virus through Woburn. Later she and other parents even talked about the possibility of an airborne virus emanating from the piles of rotting hides. In view of the fact that the virus believed to cause acquired immune deficiency syndrome (AIDS) could be related to the virus that causes human T-cell leukemia, the only human leukemia convincingly tied to a virus, and that the AIDS virus apparently may have originated in an animal gene pool in Africa, the cow hides theory is not necessarily outlandish. And a leukemia virus need not have been the only cause; a virus can well leave the human body susceptible to other assaults on the cell, say from groundwater contaminants.

Though the panel certainly made commendable and comprehensive suggestions after reviewing the situation in Woburn, it could not know that it was recommending actions that had been kicked around before and that had not enjoyed official support. For example, some of the health monitoring programs and environmental surveying recommended by the panel had been suggested in May 1980 by a group of graduate students in the Department of Urban and Environmental Policy at Tufts University who were studying the Woburn events.

The Massachusetts Cancer Registry, which the panel had called an "essential source," and on which much of future cancer incidence data would rely had almost not come into existence. Governor King of Massachusetts had vetoed the enabling legislation for it in 1979, and so FACE, particularly Bruce Young and Anne Anderson, and other groups like the League of Women Voters had to lobby intensively for its passage the next year.

And finally the major "theme" of Woburn as an environmental model community had actually first been given voice by Bruce Young in 1981 when he had said he didn't understand "why there weren't scientists crawling all over this place trying to get to the bottom of what happened here. We could be the proverbial living laboratory for finding out about chemical causes of leukemia." The suggestion that leukemic children have their blood sampled and stored for future study had also been made by Anne Anderson and Young in 1980 even before the CDC and the MDPH had confirmed the cluster existed. These samples could have been available for the 1985 panel to examine.

In a way the panel of experts in fact redefined the term *expert,* for it advanced, indeed embraced and officially endorsed, many concepts laypersons and parents had instinctively believed should be pursued all along. In the end perhaps the greatest and most lasting contribution of the expert panel was that it bestowed the crown of scientific validity on ideas that had occurred to others through available common sense.

16

Anderson et al. v. Cyrovac et al.

IN AUGUST 1985 the discovery process closed in the case of *Anne Anderson et al. v. Cyrovac*, a division of W. R. Grace Company, and other companies, charging that the poor waste disposal practices of the companies led to the contamination of groundwater, including wells G and H, and that this contamination caused the leukemias that occurred in the plaintiffs' families and in the East Woburn area.

During "discovery" each side investigates the other's case, taking a look at the cards in the hands of the opponent. The process can consume an astronomical amount of time and money and can be grueling from the plaintiff's point of view, particularly when it requires, as the Woburn case did, the detailed recounting of painful personal events in the form of depositions before attorneys representing defendants whose activities may have caused the pain but who deny responsibility.

The W. R. Grace Company, whose president, J. Peter Grace, served as a counselor to the Reagan administration on ways to eliminate what Grace isolated as wasteful federal government spending programs, refused to accept any responsibilities in Woburn for either the pollution of wells G and H or the leukemia cases.

However, Grace was no stranger to the defendant's role in water pollution litigation in the Boston area. In the town of Acton, located 22 miles west of Boston, not far from Woburn, chemical waste disposal into a landfill and several lagoons at a Grace facility allegedly led to the contamination of groundwater feeding two municipal wells. The water was found to contain trichloroethylene (TCE), dichloroethylene, methylene chloride, even benzene, and the two wells were closed in December 1978, six months before the contamination of wells G and H was discovered in Woburn. The Acton water district closed the wells, which had provided a million gallons a day or 40% of the city's water supply, and the town of Acton consequently sued the W. R. Grace Company for damages on the basis of groundwater studies that traced the contaminating plume back to the Grace site. No detailed investigations of the health picture in Acton, however, were undertaken.

When the Woburn suit against the Grace Company was filed in 1982, the company issued a press statement that said, "Grace strongly objects to the irresponsible and unjustified identification of its Woburn plant as being connected in any way with the problem outlined in the suit."

Grace cited the fact that Cyrovac did not produce chemicals but that rather it manufactured food wrapping machinery, which was true enough. However, as the EPA and DEQE traced the G and H contamination back toward a source, it put W. R. Grace under orders to sink test wells at its Cyrovac location and to report to the EPA what chemicals had been used in the Cyrovac operations. For while the Grace facility certainly did not produce chemicals such as those found in wells G and H, it did use them.

The Grace facility, a plain brick building marked with the Cyrovac logo on busy Washington Street in Woburn, looks harmless enough. Behind the plant, abutting the employee parking lot is a small, stony field that would be perfect for a sandlot baseball game except that it is now closed off by fencing with signs that say "Danger" but do not say from what. In the middle of the field is one of the test wells Grace was ordered to install to determine if contamination lay under the field. It did, and it made its way under the parking lot, newly widened town roads, even four-lane interstate highways, in a southwesterly direction toward the trapment area of wells G and H.

In response to the EPA's request for an inventory of chemicals used at the site, Grace sent a letter in February 1982. Grace claimed not to have records—users are generally not required to keep any—of exactly how it used its chemicals, only how many gallons of chemicals it had purchased. In February of 1982 Grace told the EPA it had purchased one barrel of TCE, or 55 gallons, at the plant between 1973 and 1975. But when the *Anderson et al.* suit was filed and the discovery process began, requiring Grace to answer "interrogatories"— questions in search of information that can be used as evidence in the courtroom—Grace disclosed that it had purchased and used at least four barrels of pure TCE since 1964, plus various brand name solvents like Cool Tool and Syn-Electro, which contained trichloroethylene and tetrachloroethylene, other chemicals found in

1979 in wells G and H. The chemicals were used to clean grease from machinery.

Grace also disclosed information about its disposal practices that it had not told the EPA, namely that "on a few occasions" chemicals were "spread on the ground in the area between the two drainage ditches in the rear of the plant on a sunny day for drying and evaporation." Grace called the chemicals "material from the degreaser in the machine shop" and said the company did not know what was contained in the "material" but "substances used in the degreaser from time to time included small amounts of 1,1,1-trichloroethane or tetrachloroethylene." Given the density and longevity of the solvents in question, dumping not much more than a barrel could have resulted in the readings found in wells G and H in 1979.

Grace also said that "occasionally" employees might have discarded "small amounts" of "materials" at the rear of the plant and that "it is not known what substances were so discarded." Grace further admitted that in October 1974 at least ten drums of "accumulated paint sludge" were placed in a pit dug in the area behind the building. The company said, "constituents of the paint sludge are not known, but substances used in processes yielding paint sludge as a waste by-product from time to time might have included small amounts of trichloroethylene."

The first set of Grace legal papers seemed to carefully avoid pinpointing any waste disposal to specific dates prior to 1972, particularly of TCE, the year of Jimmy Anderson's diagnosis, although Grace did admit buying TCE and using it as of 1964.

When it became known through the lawsuit that Grace had used more chemicals than it had initially admitted, FACE called a press conference in February 1983. Bruce Young pointed out that when Grace characterized the lawsuit as "irresponsible," the company had already reported to the EPA that it had used at least one barrel of TCE. And, Young noted, it was not until almost the end of 1982 that Grace provided EPA information about additional chemical use on the premises.

Release of the letters between the EPA and Grace triggered a round of speculation that the EPA had not been vigorous enough in its investigation of Grace for political reasons, perhaps because of J. Peter Grace's relationship with the president. However, the regional administrator for the EPA, Paul Keough, denied the EPA had been going slow with Grace, citing its pressure on Grace to make a "consent decree" to "spend millions of dollars to clean up the Acton aquifer." Keough reiterated though that his agency had not been given the full information about how much TCE had been in use and disposed of at the plant and said, "we might have looked at the original situation differently if we had had this information."

This prompted Senator Kennedy to write a letter to Anne Gorsuch, as head of the EPA, expressing his concern that Grace was being let off easily.

W. R. Grace then issued a statement that tended to support the "go-slow" allegations by saying, on the contrary, it was not that Grace had failed to advise the EPA fully but that the EPA had not acted on the information Grace provided. Grace said that the EPA had known about the pit used to dispose of paint sludge at the Cyrovac facilities at least a year before but had failed to inspect it. Grace added that when, as a result of the discovery process in connection with the legal suit, the company had found the new information after a search of "thousands of documents and gathering employees recollections . . . our problem was that for several weeks the EPA wouldn't meet with us to discuss this information. . . . The EPA's response . . . accuses Grace of acting in bad faith. Nothing could be further from the truth."

The second defendant in the Woburn case was the Beatrice Foods Company, which had purchased the John J. Riley Company, a tannery, in December 1978. The Riley Company, in the hands of the Riley family, had been established in 1910. The Riley property in Woburn is a few minutes' drive from the Anderson house, and the small, white clapboard office building is dwarfed by the tannery's tall smokestack reinforced with metal strapping. Beatrice sold the tannery back to the Riley family after the Woburn suit was filed, but retained all the legal liability in the matter.

The case against Beatrice was based on the groundwater studies done to trace the sources of contamination of wells G and H. As part of the process, inspections were made of the Riley plant and the 15-acre plot of undeveloped woodsy land adjacent to it. This land, Beatrice said in its interrogatories, was "used as a water source" for tanning operations. There is a private well on the property.

Tanning leather means removing hairs and stains from skins with a battery of caustic chemicals and then treating the tough hides to achieve a supple feel and an appealing look. The Riley tannery did not produce finished leather, but the hide treatment process required a veritable battery of such chemicals as dyes, waxes, resins, ethers, pigments, perfumes, soaps, salts, acids, and solvents. The process also required lots of water, both to rinse the hides and flush wastes away.

This waste water had been discharged straight into the Aberjona River until Riley received a permit to use the Woburn sewer system. Solid waste sludge, however, was left to settle through drains in the tannery floor into a settling tank underground on the property. When engineers contracted by the EPA, accompanied by a Beatrice Food Company representative, toured the Riley site, they sampled the soil of the adjacent property and water from the wells there by sampling water in the faucets connected to the wells. The Riley land is wooded and marshy and the EPA investigators noted seeing some "distressed vegetation" there, as well as several stacks of 55-gallon drums, some open, some closed, lying along the dirt road that runs through the interior of the land.

Results of the tests of the soil at Riley showed no organic volatile chemicals, other than methane, in the soil and surface water at the site, but the water from the wells was contaminated with chemicals, including TCE, in levels as high as those found in wells G and H and in the water feeding Riley's "color room" in an amount almost three times higher than that found in well G. The report also found that hazardous materials, mostly dyes, were being discharged into Woburn's municipal sewer system.

Beatrice Foods took fairly rigid refuge in what might

be called the "downstream defense," claiming that the Riley facilities lay downstream from wells G and H and thus could not have contaminated them.

Interpreting the results of the hydrological groundwater studies somewhat differently than the EPA or the plaintiffs, Beatrice argued that given the slope of the land and the groundwater flow, their property was downstream from the recharging area of the wells. The company maintained that if the water in the wells on their property was contaminated, then it too was a victim of polluted groundwater flow. Moreover, in an interview, attorney for the Beatrice Company, Jerome Facher of the Boston firm of Hale and Door, said that none of the chemicals named in the suit, including TCE, had ever been used in the tanning process and that if those chemicals were found in the Riley well water, Riley had not put them there.

However, in its answer to the interrogatories, Beatrice stopped short of denying TCE had been used, instead objecting to the question and refusing to answer the interrogatory referring to TCE use because it sought, in Beatrice's view, "information that is irrelevant and not reasonably calculated to lead to the discovery of admissible evidence."

All questions put to Beatrice about sludge disposal and whether the barrels spotted on the Riley property could have leaked and contaminated the groundwater were similarly stonewalled: "Beatrice was not aware of any solid wastes, liquids, sludge or chromium wastes being deposited on the property which is the subject of this lawsuit." Beatrice also maintained that the undeveloped land was used solely as a water source, not as a disposal site, and it claimed only that it was aware that a nearby barrel-reclaiming company, "The Whitney Barrel Company," and "persons unknown" did indeed for "years of unknown exact date leave empty barrels and debris on the grounds of the tanneries."

The questions thus became did Beatrice allow, or fail to take measures to protect against, toxic waste disposal on its property that resulted in groundwater contamination, thus polluting its own wells and wells G and H?

Also, when asked about the results of the duplicate sampling tests taken by their representative at the time EPA investigators toured the site, Beatrice said, "there were no tests conducted," directly denying the EPA description of the inspection. Beatrice also attempted to prevent Mr. John G. Riley, the original tannery owner, from giving a deposition to the plaintiffs' attorneys on the grounds that he was not party to the suit, but Riley was later ordered to answer interrogatories by the judge in the case.

Beatrice used a legal strategy of interpreting the plaintiffs' complaint very narrowly and literally. The complaint did not allege that chemicals used at the tannery caused groundwater contamination, nor that chemicals leaking from the tannery settling tanks were involved. Rather, using the only evidence available at the time, the EPA report that barrels were seen on the Riley land and that vegetation was distressed, the complaint alleged that chemicals deposited on the Riley land led to the contamination. Consequently from a strictly legal point of view, Beatrice reasoned, any questions about the settling tank process, the chemicals used in the tanning process, the sludge produced or where any of it went would be irrelevant legally. It also failed to answer any interrogatories aimed at discovering how in fact the tannery did dispose of its waste or empty the settling tank.

On this basis, Beatrice declined to answer most of the interrogatories put to it, waiting for the plaintiffs to provide some new evidence that would compel them to answer. In fact, the attorney for Beatrice, Jerome Facher, professed that when the suit was filed, Beatrice really had no idea why it had been named. He said, "there is no way we can be responsible unless there is something we don't know."

The burden of proof in civil tort litigation falls on the plaintiffs, and the Woburn plaintiffs were represented by Jan R. Schlichtmann, a lanky, confident attorney experienced in the law of medical malpractice. In fact, he was once a partner in the firm of Reed and Mulligan, the office of attorney-author Barry Reed, who wrote the best-selling book *The Verdict*, which was the basis of the popular film of the same name starring Paul Newman as a down-on-his-luck attorney who wins a major malpractice suit against a leading Boston hospital. In fact, according to the book jacket biography of Reed, in 1978 his firm indeed won one of the largest settlements for medical malpractice in Massachusetts history—$5.8 million.

Schlichtmann, who has won some major malpractice cases himself, could be said to have inherited the Woburn toxic tort case because of the legal action Donna Robbins brought to Reed and Mulligan back in 1976 when Robbie Robbins had had his sciatic nerve severed during surgery prior to his diagnosis with leukemia.

Donna Robbins filed a malpractice suit, for which she ultimately received a small amount of money, through Reed and Mulligan and became familiar with the firm. When Anne Anderson, Donna Robbins, and others decided to file a toxic tort case in connection with the leukemia incidence, Reed and Mulligan was again involved.

Schlichtmann was certainly aware of the "bigness" of the Woburn case, noting at one point, "Obviously this case has the potential to win one of the biggest verdicts in Massachusetts history" or "this kind of case will establish important new toxic tort law." But he also had serious concern about the problems of toxic waste, and as a practicing attorney in San Francisco, he helped found a branch of Trial Lawyers for Public Justice, a network of public injury lawyers who contribute their time and occasionally money to a nonprofit legal foundation that in turn funds the research necessary to bring complex scientific cases to court.

Trial Lawyers for Public Justice operates from a warren of small offices in Washington, D. C., and is headed by Anthony J. Roisman. He is regarded as a national leader of the plaintiffs bar in toxic tort litigation. Relaxed and confident as he speaks directly to a question asked, he is clearly aware that the cases he takes on have important potential for establishing legal precedents: "I wouldn't take them if they didn't." But he also believes that toxic tort litigation has a legitimate role in securing public justice given the magnitude of the toxic waste problem.

Roisman brought to private practice a close experience with public litigation of toxic waste matters. He had been chief of the Hazardous Waste Section of the United States Department of Justice, and he left, he says succinctly, "because I had no work to do." According to Roisman, during the 1981-1982 period the EPA under Anne Gorsuch, "did not refer a single hazardous waste case to the Justice Department," and cases his section wished to initiate, he says, could not move along because he could not get his superiors to push the EPA to release documents in its possession that might have been useful to the prosecution of cases. In fact when Congress sought to investigate the EPA's handling of toxic waste prosecutions, it was the Justice Department that advised Gorsuch to claim "executive privilege" and withhold the documents. Gorsuch for her part said she was told by the White House not to comply with the congressional orders. Critics in the press and Congress argued that the EPA was circling its wagons to protect toxic waste disposal violators and that it was caught in a serious conflict of interest by protecting private companies and not public environment, which was its administrative job. Ultimately Gorsuch was cited for contempt of Congress; she then dismissed her assistant for toxic waste matters, Rita M. Lavelle, and resigned herself as head of EPA in March 1983. Lavelle was later tried and convicted of perjury.

One of the issues in the Lavelle matter was whether she had written a memo criticizing her agency's chief counsel for "systematically alienating the primary constituents of this administration, the business community." Also during this period it became public that in early 1983, at the height of the crisis over whether it would respond to congressional subpoenas for documentation, the EPA had used paper shredders to dispose of some documents which had been subpoenaed—it called them "extra copies"—that could have been pertinent to toxic waste enforcement issues.

The stormy period at EPA had begun right around the time, early 1982, when the W. R. Grace Company was reporting to the EPA that it had only used one barrel of TCE and was, even according to W. R. Grace, not being vigorously investigated further.

In the absence of any program, either federally or locally funded, to compensate individuals for adverse health effects that could have been caused by exposure to toxic wastes, civil court and the tort system remained the only mechanism in place for compensating individuals for the harm they suffered and the costs they incurred. And in an era of weak enforcement by the government of government's regulations, the civil tort system was also the only avenue open to Anne Anderson and others for getting at the essential truth: how did wells G and H get contaminated, and did the wells lead to the leukemias?

But establishing truth in such cases as Woburn, given the complexities of the relevant sciences and the problems of traditional epidemiology, greatly increases the burden of proof, for instead of being able to build a neat Golden Gate across the canyon of cause and effect, plaintiffs must resort to a series of corroborating footbridges that together could add up to proof.

As the discovery process unrolled in Woburn, the W. R. Grace Company moved to sever one of the footbridges, by filing a motion of summary judgment in May 1984. This sort of legal maneuver is used in situations where one side feels there is no issue of fact to be resolved by the court or a jury—no matter in sufficient dispute to warrant a trial.

Grace's motion for summary judgment put aside for the time being the issue of whether its waste disposal practices contributed to the contamination of wells G and H. The motion instead focused on the specific but complex scientific question of whether the chemicals mentioned in the suit, specifically TCE, could actually cause leukemia. Grace contended that since the chemicals did not cause leukemia, even if they were found to have poured TCE straight into the wells, it could not be liable in the cause of the leukemia cluster. Grace said it felt entitled to a summary judgment because it felt the plaintiffs could not "make out a prima facie case that a causal nexus exists between exposure to the subject chemicals and leukemia."

Thus began the battle of the curricula vitae since in matters of dispute about scientific or technical information, in a court of law only scientific or technical experts can argue the information. To support its contention that TCE and the leukemias could not be linked, Grace filed affidavits it solicited from two experts in the field of leukemogenesis, the science of what causes leukemia, who in turn argued that in their expert opinion there was no "medically accepted evidence which would support an expert opinion on behalf of plaintiffs that it is more likely than not exposure to any of the subject chemicals caused or promoted plaintiffs' leukemia."

Thus, Grace argued, if there could be no medically accepted evidence, then any statement about cause in the trial "would amount to nothing more than rank speculation and conjecture."

The leukemia experts Grace cited, both professors at

Harvard University Medical School among other prestigious affiliations, had reviewed the medical literature
on leukemia causes and studies done on TCE. They also
included in their affidavit discussions of the extremely
complicated matter of whether data collected in animal
tests had any bearing on humans.

In fact one expert cited a study of mice that had
developed lymphosarcoma, tumors of the white cell–
producing lymph nodes, and argued that the strain of
mice used developed a high incidence of "spontaneous"
tumors, independent of whether the mice were exposed
to chemicals. The expert concluded that this particular
study illustrated "the difficulty of reliably extrapolating
results of animal studies to other species and particularly to humans until such time as the mechanisms of
leukemogenesis are better understood." Both experts
concluded that "on the basis of available evidence" TCE
was not causally related to leukemia in humans.

Grace also cited as support a 1958 case in Massachusetts in which a Supreme Court judge reversed a work-
men's compensation award on a claim that a staphylococcus infection caused the employee's leukemia. The
judge at the time had said "there is some basis for the
hypothesis that staphylococcus infection is a cause of
leukemia, but so far it is only an unproved hypothesis
which . . . may sometime be proved. This is not proof of
cause."

Perhaps deliberately, the Grace motion sought to put
the Woburn case in the context of another time. It cited
a decision made in the 1950s, when causes of cancer
were practically a complete mystery, and it cited two
albeit distinguished experts whose medical training and

professional formation had taken place in the 1930s and 1940s, prior to the generalized concern of awareness of the role of carcinogenic synthetic chemicals in human health. Given what is now known about the possible role of viruses and infectious agents and the minute changes in cell function that can take place in cancer, it may well be that the 1950s decision, if decided today, would have gone the other way. And there is a good deal more about the causes of leukemia than both affidavits reflected on which reasonable men and women could differ.

However, the Grace motion also accomplished the purpose of smoking out information, so that Grace was able to get a strong whiff of the strategy that would be used against them.

Schlichtmann, for the plaintiffs, fought science with science. He did not attempt to refute the defendant's experts, but simply introduced his own, Dr. Alan S. Levin, who, unlike the Grace experts who relied on what had been shown by the classic epidemiological model, tapped into the new frontiers of molecular epidemiology. Levin, a private physician in immunology in San Francisco and adjunct associate professor at the University of California, came to the case without the heavy prestige of Harvard on his curriculum vitae. But, he did not argue about the role of TCE in leukemia on the macro level of whether the specific chemical could lead directly to the disease on the basis of what had already been "proven." Nor did he debate whether animal data could be applied to man. Instead Levin based his affidavit on what he believed took place in the body at the subcellular level and his own clinical examination of the plaintiffs. For him the question was not whether TCE had yet been shown to cause leukemia in animals or humans. It was that TCE belonged to a group of chemicals that were known to damage cells in such a way as to leave them, possibly, able to become leukemic.

Using blood samples taken from the plaintiffs as well as examining them and reviewing their medical histories, Levin, retained by Schlichtmann in cooperation with the Massachusetts General Hospital, stated in his affidavit that the plaintiffs were all showing "abnormalities consistent with immune [system] dysregulation. There is an increased number of one subset of lymphocyte which is consistent with a compensatory response to resist the effects of a carcinogen." In other words, Levin was arguing that he had found "footprints in the snow," evidence that the plaintiffs who had not contracted leukemia had indeed suffered exposure to carcinogens, which they had, so far, successfully resisted. By implication the children in the suit, who suffered from leukemia, had been unsuccessful in the same resistance attempt.

Levin described the cell and spoke of how TCE and other halogenated hydrocarbons, the group of chemicals to which TCE belongs, "have been shown to cause damage to DNA in human lymphocytes and the expression of endogenous tumor viruses. These are the major mechanisms which contribute to the development of human leukemia." Levin also cited studies which showed that TCE had damaged the human liver, "thereby reducing this organ's ongoing capacity to neutralize toxic substances which cause diseases such as cancer and leukemia."

In other words, where the Grace attorneys had focused on whether the chemicals in question had yet actually been proved to induce human leukemia, the plaintiffs' attorneys focused on whether the action of these chemicals on the individual cell could be ruled out as a cause of leukemia. It put the courtroom in the laboratory, and it shifted the axis of the case from past to present and future.

The Levin affidavit, the study done by the Harvard biostatistics department, plus the CDC and MDPH studies which showed that a cluster existed and that it could be statistically related to the wells led Schlichtmann to ask that the motion for summary judgment be dismissed because there were still issues in dispute.

The judge in the case agreed. On July 25, 1984, he wrote in his opinion dismissing the Grace motion, "Since the complex factual issue of causation is a subject of heated dispute in this case, summary judgement is clearly inappropriate." With this the case jumped up a level, establishing that the argument would be not only about how wells G and H became contaminated but also about what changes in the human cell could have added up to the death of Jimmy Anderson and the other children.

Dr. Levin's statements were not irrefutable, of course. And they were based on allergy research, not human leukemia research directly. However, like the Harvard study, Levin's work was, at the least, intellectually provocative. From a legal standpoint it is a bonanza for attorneys in that it fills a gap long missing in toxic tort litigation—physical evidence of toxic exposure. If one could no longer find the chemical TCE in the bodies of the plaintiffs, one could perhaps see its tracks. Levin's footprints in the snow could be argued as proving that enough TCE did indeed enter the bodies of those in the case, marking their blood cells and their immune system. Therefore it followed that the children who died also suffered this exposure and were marked in the form of lethal disease. It also followed that those who have not yet contracted leukemia remained nevertheless at higher risk of the disease, that is, more susceptible to it than other people not similarly exposed.

Levin's evidence built on the basic theory of immunity, that when the body is exposed to any foreign substance, an antigen, the immune system springs into action to neutralize it, the very process scientists mimic to track DNA damage using adduct antibodies.

Levin and others in the field extend the theory of immunity to include pollutants, which could stimulate the immune system to get rid of them just like a germ would. Evidence of stimulation of the immune system, Levin argued, could be seen in the plaintiff's blood, through such readings as increased levels of eosinophils and T-cell lymphocytes, two forms of white blood cells directly involved in the immune system, as well as in depressed levels of blood proteins, which are also important in regulating immune reactions. These reactions are similar to what is seen in patients who, for example, come in contact with a substance to which they are allergic.

The theory that chemicals in the air and water in Woburn entered the bodies of the children would be consistent with rashes and skin outbreaks suffered by some of the children, in particular Robbie Robbins, and the issue of why some children got leukemia and others didn't might well have had to do with age and strength of the immune system at the time.

At least since the mid-1970s there have been studies suggesting that immune factors may be involved in certain cancers, including one study in 1973 in which twelve members of a family of American Indians all developed stomach cancers, but the family members without cancer had defects in cell-mediated immunity, the same set of body responses cited by Levin in the case of the Woburn families.

Evidence of future risk from cancer and other disease possibly due to immune system deficiencies makes the toxic waste issue even more explosive legally, since increased susceptibility to disease has been established as a damage for which plaintiffs can be compensated under tort law. In the case of Jackson Township, New Jersey, for example, $8.2 million of the $17 million verdict was to be applied to pay for a medical examination for each and every plaintiff every year for the rest of their lives. Dr. Susan Daum, an expert in acute effects of exposures to toxic substances such as asbestos and pesticides, argued strongly in the trial that anyone exposed to the contaminated water should be examined medically every year. She said later in a telephone interview, "I felt then and still do that people suffering such exposures should have the money to pay for a sophisticated medical workup each year that would surpass what is ordinarily available to a regular doctor, given that in the next few years there will be a very big change in what we can do about cell surface markers and detection of cancer."

In fact, while the Jackson Township verdict was being

appealed and about fifteen months after the decision, a three-year-old boy in the Legler neighborhood, who lived in one of the eight houses with the mysterious incidence of kidney disease and at least one rare kidney cancer, was diagnosed with a rare neuroblastoma, a brain cancer, of which there had been no sign during the trial.

The Woburn case demonstrated clearly that legal strategies can be fixed in time, while science is dynamic. For example, the Grace motion which argued that TCE was not considered a leukemogen failed to refer to a paper that appeared the very month the motion was filed, May 1984, in the *American Journal of Industrial Medicine*. Written by a team of epidemiologists from the University of North Carolina and the Georgetown University Medical School, the report was entitled "An Evaluation of the Associations of Leukemia and Rubber Industry Solvent Exposures." It found that whereas benzene, the most well-accepted chemical leukemogen, had been previously largely associated with myelocytic leukemia, it also appeared to have an association with lymphocytic leukemia as well. But perhaps most significant was what the study turned up about solvents other than benzene: "The associations with lymphocytic risk observed for a number of solvents, most notably carbon tetrachloride and carbon disulfide, were stronger than those detected for benzene." TCE was among the number of solvents positively associated with lymphocytic leukemia in workers in the rubber industry, though its association was dramatically less obvious than that of carbon tetrachloride. However, carbon tetrachloride is not generally accepted as a leukemogen either.

With the motion for a summary judgment dismissed, discovery continued, and more of the historical tableau of the case was sketched in. It was confirmed, for example, through depositions taken from Grace employees, that the Cyrovac facility had little or no plan for disposal of toxic wastes in the 1960s and early 1970s. The chief pollution control officer for Cyrovac said in depositions that during this period his preferred method for eliminating wastes at the plant was to let them "evaporate into the air." Another employee stated that he had recommended to the company that it hire a "legal" hauler to take the waste away in barrels rather than have the workers simply pour it on the ground in the back of the plant, which was the practice at the time. He stated he did not know whether haulers were ever called, but shortly after his recommendation, he said, the company began burying barrels of waste behind the facility.

It also came to light that in 1974 an official from Grace Corporate headquarters had sent a memo to various Grace divisions, including Cyrovac, that TCE should no longer be used in the facilities because of its carcinogenic potential and impending legislation that might affect companies using the chemical.

In 1981 the same officer had failed to file required reports with the Metropolitan District Commission, into whose sewers Cyrovac was discharging wastes, that 400 gallons of metal cleaners and 100 gallons of metal solvents had been disposed of into the sewer system.

The Riley tannery had also had its share of past environmental problems. As early as 1951 it had been told by the Office of the Massachusetts Commissioner of Public Health that wastes from the tannery which were being allowed to overflow onto the ground "from a distribution box in the tannery sewer line leading to your settling tanks" were also reaching the Aberjona River and the metropolitan sewer system, contrary to law.

Also in 1974, two cases of employee cancer were investigated by the Riley Company, but an internal memo said because none of the dyes to which the workers were believed to have been exposed were known to be carcinogenic and because the employees had worked for the Riley Company fewer years than the fifteen cited as "the incubation period" for cancer, that "it is unlikely that the exposure which has caused their cancer was had" at the Riley Company and "if the employees were exposed to carcinogenic dyes at previous employments, it would be those previous employers and not [the Riley Company] that would be responsible."

The long history of poor waste disposal and general environmental practices in the Woburn area was cited by both Beatrice and Grace as evidence that their own facilities should not be the focus of any suit in the 1980s. According to Mark Stoler, an in-house attorney for the W. R. Grace Company, "the town should have written that aquifer off long ago."

As of summer 1985 the town of Woburn had not instigated legal action against companies for contaminating the groundwater, but the possibility could not be foreclosed. And information continued to come in. For example, when the EPA discovered that contamination emanating from the Interstate Uniform Services, a uniform cleaning company operating in Woburn, might also have contaminated wells G and H, they were added to the suit filed by the Woburn families.

While the physical evidence on the extent of the groundwater contamination was being collected, the defendants continued making legal arguments. W. R. Grace and Beatrice Foods filed a joint motion to dismiss parts of the case in early 1985 on the grounds that even if the exposure to wells G and H had caused the leukemias of Jimmy Anderson, Robbie Robbins, and Michael Zona, their claims should be dismissed because more than the three years stipulated in the state's statute of limitations had expired between the "injury" which caused the death and the suit, working ahead from the dates of diagnosis. The motion also argued that parents could not sue for compensation for emotional distress claiming that the emotional distress had been brought on by Dr. Levin's assertion that they were at future risk of disease, not from having watched their children die.

Schlichtmann counter-argued that the law had been "tolling" on his clients' behalf until they could know their children may have suffered injury, namely May 1979 when it was discovered that the well water had been contaminated. A suit therefore had to be filed within three years of that date, which it was. He also maintained that compensation for emotional distress in the Woburn case was supported by the laws in Massachusetts, challenging the defendants' interpretations of that law. A trial was not expected before late fall of 1985.

The case was certainly complicated, and one wonders what would have been the defendants' legal strategy if it had been more clear-cut, for example, if benzene had been the only chemical found in the wells and if all the leukemias had been of the type generally agreed to be associated with benzene.

Between environmental epidemiology and the law

there are many ways to make an argument. For example, in May 1983 Dr. Philip Cole of the University of Alabama was retained by Epidemiology Resources, Inc., a private firm, to conduct a study for the Shell Oil Company at one of its refineries in Wood River, Illinois. The Shell Oil Company wanted to establish what the leukemia rate was among workers there and to see if there was a relationship with benzene exposure, in connection with regulations for benzene exposure then being debated by the Occupational Safety and Health Administration (OSHA).

Cole's report, dated July 6, 1983, stated that indeed between 1973 and 1982 there had been a fourfold increase in risk of death from leukemia. The total of fourteen cases represented an excess of 7.6 cases over what would be expected, which Cole called "highly statistically significant." Of the fourteen cases observed, eight were of the myelocytic type, the type of leukemia most closely associated with benzene.

Cole also wrote, "The fact that virtually the entirety of the excess cases, that is 6 of 7.6, are of the AML (acute myelocytic leukemia) form is unequivocal evidence of a genuinely increased risk of death from this specific condition."

Cole also wrote, "I would strongly recommend to Shell that the present findings be prepared for publication in a scientific journal. Even in their present form the data provide a strong link between benzene and AML." Cole also suggested there be further research to see if the level of benzene exposures correlated with the leukemia cases, if the workers with leukemia suffered the highest benzene exposures. He wrote that if these

studies were positive, "the resultant findings would become among the most important in the entire medical
literature on the causes of leukemia."

The proposed research was undertaken in a second
phase. The study sought to quantify the levels of exposure according to job description, say extractor foreman
compared to machinist. A benzene-exposed job was defined as one "if the unit in which the job was located
contained a stream with benzene in excess of 5% concentration or if the job involved the 'open' handling of
substances containing more than 1% benzene." A yearly
dose of benzene was estimated based on the tasks performed and the frequency of the tasks and the intensity
of the exposure with each task.

The results were collected in a follow-up report by
Cole and an associate, and there were no AML cases
found among the jobs believed to be of highest exposure.
However, the report said "there is a suggestion in the
data that the cases, especially the AML cases, were more
heavily exposed than were the controls." The study concluded "the study has produced no distinctly positive
result, not even for benzene, and the reason for the excess among the refinery workers remains unexplained."
Dr. Cole himself said, to the *Wall Street Journal* in February 1985 and in a subsequent telephone interview, "At
present, I remain of the persuasion that the most likely
cause of the leukemias is the benzene." On the matter
of the inconclusive results of the exposure level studies,
he said, "Common sense tells me it's benzene, but you
can't establish scientific fact on that."

According to George Machino, vice-president of Local
525 of the International Union of Operating Engineers,

the workers in the refinery did not know the full results of Cole's research until they read about it in press accounts. In fact, according to Machino, while the research was being conducted, the union was not aware of exactly why the research was being done. Because the workers were "blind" to ensure they would not introduce bias into the results, neither were they told that the deaths from leukemia at the plant had been higher than expected. Nor, Machino said, were the workers ever told about the extent of the scientific literature which said that benzene was a known leukemogen.

The union was told by Shell that Dr. Cole had strongly suspected benzene as a cause even though his study of exposure levels did not categorically link it with the illnesses. Benzene, after all, is one of the few accepted human leukemogens that has not been conclusively linked to leukemia in laboratory animals. Thus its carcinogenic behavior is known to be unpredictable if widely accepted.

Machino said, "The company sent another doctor out to talk with us, but he said there was no proven link between leukemia and benzene, so we accepted it. He made a heck of an argument that there was no link. Who are we, not having the credentials or background, to dispute it?"

According to Machino, the union and the workers were not given a complete copy of Cole's reports, "only a summary which played down the connection with benzene." When Shell representatives were questioned about why they had not provided the full report, the company said it was because it had not been asked by the workers to do so.

17

The Flawed Net of Detection

AMAZINGLY, even the most sophisticated data system in place in the United States as of July 1985 would be unable on its own to notice a cluster like Woburn's as it was happening. It would still take an alert individual to get the first hint of a problem—real or fluke. And only if that individual succeeded in interesting public authorities would a cluster be investigated further.

Cancer registries were intended to monitor trends in the disease, and their concept is not new. In 1935 Connecticut became the first state to establish a cancer registry, when a group of physicians became concerned, after looking at rudimentary data based on death certificates, that New Haven suffered the highest rate of cancer deaths of any city in the United States. The rate had more than doubled there—from 66 per 100,000 persons to 180 per 100,000—between 1900 and 1934.

So with a $10,000 appropriation and large record books filled in by clerks using fountain pens, the registry began. The increased rate of death in New Haven was ultimately attributed to the growing role of the city as a treatment center for cancer cases.

Few states have cancer incidence registries, and the only national overview source of cancer statistics, the

SEER program, extrapolates a national picture of cancer incidence from data collected from a percentage of the population. And in 1985, setting up a computerized registry can cost roughly a quarter of a million dollars.

But detecting clusters, even through the best registries, does not mean a cluster and a potential cause will be put together. A mortality registry will not pick up a cluster until the people who comprise it have died, and by then, causes would be doubly difficult to reconstruct. And most incidence registries attribute a diagnosis to the town where the patients live at the time of diagnosis. In practice this system means that if one drinks water contaminated with carcinogens in one town and then moves to another and develops leukemia, one's leukemia will not be attributed to the town where the causative agent may have been. In short, most registries cannot grasp the full potential size of a cluster unless all the cases are within the boundaries of a county or town.

In Woburn this led to a number of cases being "disputed" by FACE. For example, a child who lived in Woburn prior to diagnosis and then moved to nearby Winchester is not counted by the Massachusetts Cancer Registry as a Woburn case, regardless of where the child spent the latency period. Neither is a child who moved to Augusta, Georgia, whose father, when he read about the discovery of the well contamination and the confirmation of the leukemia cluster, reported his daughter's leukemia to Bruce Young to make him aware of the case. But she still is not considered a Woburn case, even though she spent the latency period living in East Woburn, where she probably was exposed to water in wells

G and H. The "disputed" cases mean that—based on data Anne Anderson or Bruce Young track down unofficially—the total number of cases in Woburn, old and "new," is higher than can ever be officially recognized by the CDC or the MDPH.

Not only do cancer registries fail to account for a person's moving from one town to another, a "first cut" of the data would be unlikely to pick up a neighborhood cluster, which may consist of a very few cases statistically significant in terms of their own small geography. Such a tiny grouping might well disappear when lumped in with data from the larger town. For example, a cancer incidence registry would not generally pick up several cases of cancer on one block—which may be amazingly unusual—unless the incidence in the town is high enough to call attention to the town, and unless the attention called to the town would lead someone to investigate further who might then happen to find out some of the cases were on the same block. In other words, how you cut the data depends on what you are looking for, but what you are looking for depends on what you already know about the incidence of cases. Also a cancer registry may not "kick out" its data every year, so that a pocket of disease may take a few years to attract attention.

The main drawback to registries by town or county is that they can miss clusters which may have in common an exposure to an environmental carcinogen that crosses town barriers. Just as the Woburn odor does not honor town limits, neither do ambient pollutants in air and certainly in groundwater. In other words, even the best cancer registry has no effective means of relating cancer cases to possible environmental culprits—registries deal in numbers, not cause.

Registries are a start, but the national system for gathering cancer information is simply too crude to pick up subtleties like the leukemia cases in East Woburn, unless nudged by sharp-eyed individuals. In that this nudging is the only way that the pockets of disease possibly related to environmental contamination can come to light, a general sequence of events tends to occur, regardless of what community is involved: Usually a reasonably thoughtful, untrained person with a good memory who is predisposed to have faith in institutions and authority has a hunch based on common sense, puts it before an official body, and gets little or no action. That person might give up or might continue gathering information and even eventually secure some official notice. But almost always, the searches—by individuals or institutions—have a Christopher Columbus quality about them. Looking for India, the explorers almost always find something else of more immediate importance.

Such was the case of a woman for the purposes of this book referred to as Mrs. Andrea Garpaski. She lived on Round Lake, near Alden Hills and New Brighton, Minnesota, both suburbs of Minneapolis. Requesting her real name not be used, she said, "I've already had more exposure on this than I ever intended or wanted."

Across from her home stands the Twin Cities Army Munitions Plant, which is owned by the federal government and operated by several contractors, including the Federal Cartridge Corporation, the Minnesota Mining and Manufacturing Company, and the Honeywell Corporation.

When the plant was under construction in 1941, New Brighton, which in 1985 had 23,500 people, was a hamlet of 700. But during the construction of the munitions plant the population doubled almost overnight, to the delight of local merchants. And some of the $30 million the government was spending to build the plant was trickling down to those who built housing for the plant's personnel and construction workers and to those who supplied groceries and other provisions needed when a large installation is in the making. An article in a local newspaper reported in 1941 that "Placid New Brighton is stirring from its Rip Van Winkle slumber . . . it is becoming a boom town." Some of the townspeople, accustomed to other big enterprises that had come and gone like meat packing plants, a pickle plant, a cannery, and an ironworks, were cautious about the latest burst of mercantile activity. According to the press report, "how long the present boom will remain, none can guess, but there are many in the town who are optimistic, believing it will continue on a thriving scale for a generation at least."

The plant was completed and was fully operating during World War II, the Korean War, and the Vietnam War, although it is possible that some munitions were produced on the site as early as the 1930s.

In 1971 Mrs. Garpaski noticed that the surface of the lake at various points along the shore line would occasionally look "whitish and scummy." She had heard old timers in the area talk about raw sewage going into the lake from the arsenal and about "arsenal pipes," even how "the lake sometimes steamed when acid from the arsenal pipes hit the raw sewage."

Since Mrs. Garpaski thought her drinking water

came from wells that collected lake drainage and since she had a new baby at the time, she reported the unsightly water to the Minnesota Pollution Control Agency (MPCA). She remembers being told by the clerk who took her call that "nothing was going into the lake." She accepted the assurance on faith.

A little bit later, however, she noticed the whitish water again and again phoned the agency. This time she says she was told that the agency was new and underfunded and did not have a person on staff who could come out and sample the lake water. Undaunted, Mrs. Garpaski offered to collect the sample herself if the agency would perform the necessary tests. Of course certain types of water sampling must be done according to strict procedures to avoid contamination in the sampling process, but Mrs. Garpaski was not told. Her sampling method proved to be irrelevant. When she reached the agency with her jar of milky water, the clerk to whom she had been talking exclaimed, "My God, I don't even have to test that water to know there is something wrong with it." The agency representative assured her he would look into the quality of Round Lake, and Mrs. Garpaski thought her involvement in the problem was over.

Not long after, the Arden Hills Recreational Commission, of which Mrs. Garpaski was a member, was invited to tour the arsenal property because, she says, the commission had been told the government was considering donating some arsenal land to be used as a park. "As we toured," she recalls, "our guide was telling us how 'someone on the lake had turned them in,' and they now had to have men on duty around the clock to figure out what they were putting in the lake." Mrs. Garpaski did not let on that she had been the instigator, but she was secretly pleased that action had been taken on the basis of her complaint. She says now with a touch of irony in her voice, "I felt everything was taken care of." Ten years passed until 1981.

By then it was the post–Love Canal era, and the Superfund law had been enacted. Mrs. Garpaski had been reading articles about chemicals finding their way untreated into the Mississippi River, and she said, "I flashed back to our own lake and when we had had our own problem." She decided to find out the results of her original water sample with the intention of taking another one for comparison. When she called the MPCA, no record of any 1971 sampling could be found. The only file located contained a slip of paper with Mrs. Garpaski's telephone number and the words "anonymous caller," although Mrs. Garpaski had given the agency her full name and address.

Mrs. Garpaski, her concern rising, decided she would undertake to have the water in her home sampled with or without the MPCA's help. She made a number of phone calls to find a water-sampling service to get estimates for the job. But she was told the testing would be less expensive if she could specify in advance the substances for which she wanted the water tested. Stumped, she decided to call the army in Washington to see if she could learn what sorts of chemicals were usually used in munitions production. One call led to another as it tends to do, and she was put in touch with the United States Army's Hazardous Waste Group. "I was told their sole purpose was to keep track of what arsenals had dumped." She learned that the group had inspected the arsenal, that its report was not a classified document, and that surely the arsenal itself could provide a copy. But when Mrs. Garpaski phoned her friend who had given the recreation commission tour, he said he had no knowledge of the report, and according to Mrs. Garpaski, he "threatened that if I tried to get it, I'd be put onto an FBI list."

Mrs. Garpaski is not a subversive woman. She is an intelligent, calm citizen who describes herself as patriotic. The thought that she might be put on an FBI list for requesting an unclassified report simply did not make sense to her. She insisted. Finally the arsenal relinquished a copy of the "Installation Assessment of Twin Cities Army Ammunition Plant, Report No. 129," which was published in October 1978. Looking for India, Mrs. Garpaski had discovered vastly unexpected information.

The report declared its purpose was to identify contamination on the arsenal grounds and "assess the potential for contaminant migration beyond the installation boundary." The report described abandoned sewer lines that contained potentially explosive contamination, leaching pits for disposing of lead-contaminated waste water, pits for burning explosives, solvents, and cyanide waste; two pits where "large quantities of chemicals" had been buried in the 1940s; and one entire building "suspected of being contaminated with radioactive wastes from past installation activities." Based on a tour of the facility, available written records, and one monitoring well sunk in 1976, the study concluded "there is no indication of contaminants migrating beyond the installation boundaries from past manufacturing and disposal operations."

It did not seem likely to Mrs. Garpaski that underground wastes would stop at a fence line, and so she again called the MPCA. But she was still most concerned about possible leaking radioactivity from the abandoned sewage lines, not realizing the implications of the presence of the other chemicals. She offered to accompany the MPCA on a tour of the arsenal and the lake area and urged them to get a copy of the arsenal report before making the tour. Representatives of the MPCA toured the arsenal alone, but when Mrs. Garpaski again telephoned to learn what they had found, she was told there was no radioactive leakage at the arsenal. "What about building 538?" she recalls asking, wondering how an arsenal that had one completely contaminated edifice could not be leaking radioactivity. She says she was told, "Well we couldn't tour it because it was locked up." She asked again whether the MPCA had secured a copy of the arsenal report and was again told the agency was in the process of getting a copy.

At this point, Mrs. Garpaski had reached a limit of sorts. She says now looking back, "Generally I am a peaceable woman, a mother, and I don't have the time or the energy to get involved in fights. But I felt I was just being humored. This was a fight, and I am not really a fighting person. But it was my children that I was worried about; I was concerned about the water they were drinking, and I simply could not believe that books such as the one I had gotten weren't probably on library shelves all around the country. Wasn't anybody reading them?"

Disappointed and frustrated with the response of the MPCA, she telephoned a local television station. A crew visited her house and the lake and borrowed her copy of the report. The evening news broke the story that the arsenal contained toxic wastes. The next day Mrs. Garpaski received a call from a representative of the MPCA, who assured her the agency had gotten the report and was looking into the matter.

The MPCA did not find the India of radioactive wastes in the lake water samples. But when the MPCA tested private wells that drew on groundwater in the area of the arsenal, it did find a dazzling array of organic volatile chemicals. Then the Minnesota Board of Health tested public wells. Both private and public water showed high concentrations of dichloroethane, trichloroethane, dichloroethylene, and trichloroethylene (TCE), practically the identical menu of contaminants found in Woburn in wells G and H. Moreover later tests showed that the contaminating plume covered more than 18 square miles in area, fouling the aquifer that supplied 75% of the groundwater used in the area.

All municipal wells in New Brighton, Arden Hills, and the neighboring town of St. Anthony were closed. Subsequently the city of New Brighton sued the army, the Department of Defense, the Federal Cartridge Corporation, the Honeywell Corporation, and other defendants for $8 million to cover the costs it incurred in drilling the new wells. Several private suits were also initiated.

Chemicals found in the wells, such as TCE, were indeed used on the arsenal grounds in great quantities. However, the army denied that its practices contaminated the municipal groundwater, even though the groundwater within the arsenal grounds was so contaminated the army provided bottled water for all its employees. The army continued to maintain that on the basis of its interpretation of underwater groundwater flow, the contamination it generated was "contained on the arsenal property," and the likelier source of municipal contamination was "off-post," such as local landfills, a tanker yard, an oil refinery, and a solvent recycler.

As of spring 1985 the wells feeding Mrs. Garpaski's house showed only "trace" amounts of the TCE and other chemicals, but a neighbor had readings as high as 300 ppb, which is even higher than wells G and H in Woburn. Municipal readings were as high as 270 ppb.

The army spent roughly $5 million on studies of groundwater flow and began cleanup operations of the arsenal site, which could cost as much as $21 million, along with the Honeywell Company and others who lease arsenal property. But the army has refused to participate in rehabilitating the aquifer outside the arsenal. The MPCA received a $2 million Superfund grant to study the full extent of the off-site contamination and what can be done about it and has said it believed the arsenal to be the major source of the problem.

In the meantime the Garpaskis installed a water cooler in their kitchen and began drinking only bottled water. Mrs. Garpaski was not angry, just somewhat dismayed: "I do not understand why my government is willing to spend millions to prove that it did not contaminate my water. If they would just give us water I can be sure is safe. . . . All I ask is that they all put their minds to cleaning up this problem."

Mrs. Garpaski reflected on what it took to secure action on the waste problem: "I have always had complete faith. I always was for apple pie and flag waving and still am, and I have always felt I had nothing to worry about because my government was there looking out for me."

Also, her concern for anonymity derived in no small measure from the fact that for the first time in her life, in 1984, she was subjected to an extensive—what she feels is unnecessarily extensive—tax audit by the Internal Revenue Service. She was self-employed and operated an antique doll business and had never before had a tax problem. She said, "Everytime I feel I am getting paranoid, I think back to the time I was told that asking for an unclassified report might get me on an FBI list."

As for taking credit for standing firm, Mrs. Garpaski says, "I did what I did for my children. They were conceived on that water and I don't want them to have problems down the line. I don't want any special credit for doing what seemed like the only thing do do."

While it is obvious that public agencies may wish to shield their sources in public documents, wording on internal MPCA documents gives the impression that it was an early agency initiative, and not a long history of individual citizen nudging, that unveiled the extent of the arsenal contamination. For example, a memo from the Regulation Compliance Section of the MPCA to its executive director in May 1981 says "The Division of Water . . . recently visited the Twin City Army Ammunition Plant in response to area citizen concerns about possible sanitary sewer overflows of radioactive wastewater into Round Lake. These fears appear to be unfounded. However, the Division of Water Quality . . . obtained a report titled, 'Installation Assessment of Twin Cities.' " And so a long saga became a short opening paragraph to a report on contamination of water supplies for roughly 60,000 people. And the true story is not generally discussed, even known.

John Drawz, the attorney who was litigating the action against the arsenal on behalf of the city of New Brighton, when asked how the MPCA became involved in the issue, said, "I would not care to characterize how they came to be doing it." A clerk in the New Brighton engineer's office said, "because the army's involved, nobody is talking much, but the story I heard is that the Department of Natural Resources wanted to drain the lake to make the area more habitable, and the residents did not want the water level changed, and so they used the Freedom of Information Act and got a document that stopped the process."

18

The Sentinel Disease

TOXIC CONTAMINATION of the New Brighton area groundwater brought a next tier of problems into view—possible health effects among the thousands of people who had been using the water. Even before she knew that the groundwater was contaminated with chemicals, Mrs. Garpaski says she had noticed that the children in the Round Lake area seemed to complain often about headaches. Some families in the area complained of frequent stomach disorders.

The problem of how to evaluate the possible effects on public health of the extensive water contamination at New Brighton was so intimidating in scope that the Minnesota State Legislature granted $95,000 to the state department of health just to see if a credible, useful epidemiological study was feasible. An epidemiologist with the department of health, explaining the reason for the feasibility study, said, "We want to see if we can do a study that will not end up being so criticized that it will not have any meaning. These studies are very hard to do, and we want to plan ours well or not do one at all." Of course, the longer the state waited to look for effects, the less likely it would be to find those that could be detected in blood and tissue analyses, like kidney and liver dysfunction. Since the contamination came to light in 1981 and most of the residents had therefore begun drinking bottled water or had had their houses connected to the new municipal system, it is possible that subtle clinical changes in their bodies—cellular liver and kidney damage—might no longer be detectable in tests by the time the tests were conducted.

Cancer clusters would be just as difficult to locate. Minnesota has no cancer incidence registry, for example, and so determining whether there are increases in cancer cases would require a hospital-by-hospital check, and a good number of New Brighton area cases would probably be diagnosed in Minneapolis, where there are a number of large hospitals. Also, since the contamination may well have begun in the 1930s or certainly as early as the 1940s, searching for cancer cases would mean poring over decades of hospital admissions records.

The state did have some statistics available on cancer deaths, but they were not computerized, and so a search for mortality clusters would also require an extensive investment of money and manpower. Collecting data on other health problems, such as birth defects or chronic neurological dysfunction, which might cause headaches, would also be difficult. Headache is a symptom, not a disease, and quantifying the number of times children had headaches would be virtually impossible. A good place to start would have been to give all the children in the Round Lake area a comprehensive physical examination to collect information that might be compared with information collected later, but this approach was not suggested.

And so if the children in the Round Lake area suffered headaches or other damage because of their contact with contaminated water, even the most feasible epidemiological study would be unable to describe or find it.

In addition to this difficulty of determining adverse health effects on individuals, before the groundwater studies were complete, it would also not be possible to say exactly which residential areas were more closely affected. Given the veritable soup of contaminants found on the arsenal and the potential for other contamination from "off-site sources," even if an epidemiological study were to detect a disease pattern or even a bona fide cluster too big to be attributable to chance, the prospect of linking the illnesses to specific contaminants is extremely remote.

And so, all things being equal, if water contamination in the New Brighton area had had, or continued to have, deleterious effects on the health of residents, any study intended to discover this would probably be unable to draw a firm conclusion, not least of all because it was undertaken long after the fact. And though a feasibility study certainly anticipates that bind, it cannot eliminate it.

This proverbial catch-22 applies to every toxic waste site, indeed every potential locus of environmental contamination, in the United States. The problem was significant enough to be noted by the Universities Associated for Research and Education in Pathology, which published a comprehensive review of all epidemiological studies done on health effects at toxic waste sites as of spring 1985. The report noted that of the 546 waste sites at the time on the EPA priority cleanup list, only sixty-three had been studied for attendant health effects. The report concluded that while there was "little scientific evidence that chemical disposal sites have had serious effects on the health of populations living near them," it emphasized that all the health studies available had been done long after environmental culprits may have fled.

All around the country mysterious pockets of illness like Woburn's have cropped up, and they touch virtually every American industry, including the new high-technology enterprises of Silicon Valley in California on which a good deal of the future economic health of the country depends. The computer industry, however, in turn depends on the use of highly toxic gases and chemicals for the production of the tiny but all-important semiconductor microchips that are the brain cells of computers. In fact, in 1983 in California 41% of the documented cases of occupational systemic poisoning were in the semiconductor industry.

Wastes in the factories are disposed of outside them, and in 1983 500 residents of the Silicon Valley sued the Fairchild Camera and Instrument Company and other companies, alleging that the companies' waste disposal practices, including the overtaxing of an underground tank with wastes that then bubbled and seeped into the residents' water system, led to contamination of their water supply with toxic solvents, including TCE, 1,1,1-trichloroethane, xylene, acetone, and isopropyl alcohol. The residents had experienced high rates of congenital heart defects in children, as well as various cancers. A part of the legal defense was that the chemicals were not scientifically accepted to be carcinogenic. It was a replay of the Woburn events. And it wasn't alone.

In 1982 a mother in the small community of Belgrade, Maine, noticed that there seemed to be an unusual number of leukemia cases among children in the town. And when state health officials looked into the incidence, the mother was correct—five cases when two would have been expected—a handful among the community of 2,000. The increase was statistically significant, and the Maine Department of Health tested water in the homes of the victims for radon, a radioactive gas known to be common in Maine groundwater. They also tested soil samples along the roadside because parents suspected that herbicide spraying to keep weeds from the asphalt might have had something to do with the leukemias. According to Dr. Gregory Bogdan, assistant director of the Health Bureau's Division of Disease Control, "we found no explanation for the cluster," and of the residue pesticide that was found, "we don't think that was involved because there is no known association with leukemia."

Without having any environmental measurements going back in time, the health bureau's report in January 1983 concluded, "the absence of any discernible environmental risk factor present among Belgrade's population increases the likelihood that the observation of leukemia cases among Belgrade residents reflects the chance occurrence of high-risk individuals residing in the same area rather than the results of exposure to some external environmental risk factor." The fact that the individuals' high-risk status may have derived from some immunological damage brought on a number of years ago could not be explored.

Rebecca Parr, a housewife in Friendly Hills, Colorado, was among a group of residents whose homes were discovered in the fall of 1984 to have been built on bentonite, a soil with high clay content that expands when wet. The practical effect is that walls split and crack, nails pop out of walls, and sections of a house rise while other parts sink. The site should never have been used for a development, and the neighborhood had practically no resale value. The residents' only remedy was to sue the developer who built and sold the homes. Mrs. Parr, however, also noticed, in talking with neighbors about the housing problems, that a number of families complained of enlarged spleens, headaches, and seizures among their children. A little more digging turned up a cancer here and there, what has in fact emerged as an elevated incidence of cancer, in general among children, though not of the same type. One little boy was diagnosed with a rare neuroblastoma, the same sort of tumor diagnosed in Jackson Township, New Jersey.

In searching for cause, Mrs. Parr was inclined to suspect the water but was told by local water authorities the Friendly Hills water supply had no problems. But in 1984 news broke of heavy contamination filtering into the water supply system of Denver at large, possibly from a site owned by the Martin Marietta Company, which provides components for the NASA space shuttle. Water then tested in Friendly Hills did show heavy metal contamination, and there was some geological dispute as to whether the community would have been receiving water from the aquifer known to be contaminated with organic solvents.

As of spring 1985 there was no conclusive finding at Friendly Hills, and Mrs. Parr commented, somewhat resignedly, "The health authorities don't seem to want to talk much about this, and I don't have a scientific background. Our water has not been routinely tested. It seems to me that taking a test just once won't tell you very much. But I don't know. . . . I don't have any particular training in all this. Just a concern." According to Mrs. Parr, she was also feeling some opposition to her investigations among her neighbors. "What we come up against is people getting mad when you start talking publicly to try to get something done. They see it only as their real estate value going down."

Of course it is important to remember that a certain amount of clustering of any disease will indeed occur through chance alone. And it is possible that a certain number of clusters near a suspicious environmental condition—a toxic waste site, radioactivity in the air, solvents in the water—will also be casual artifacts of the odds. But what is remarkable is that there is yet no way to distinguish one from the other. And what seems even more remarkable is that epidemiology still seems bent on looking only for what is already known, particularly when large economic factors are at stake.

A particular case in point involves an acknowledged 15% increase above statewide average rates for breast cancer among women who live in Nassau County, New York. Breast cancer, of course, is closely associated with life-style factors, such as diet, ethnic origin, and socio-economic status, as well as age, a woman's childbearing and hormonal history, and history of breast cancer in the family. Breast cancer, according to Dr. Robert Niebling of the Nassau County Board of Health, is known to be common among middle-aged affluent women of

Jewish background. Nassau County has a high proportion of women residents who fall into this category.

Nassau County and adjoining Suffolk County also
have, however, an extensive problem of groundwater
contamination due in large part to residential septic
tank runoff and pesticides used for lawns and other or-
namental gardening, as well as for the few remaining
agricultural enterprises.

However, the study embarked upon by Nassau County was designed only to investigate for a relationship
between the cancer pattern and the known risk factors,
on the idea that if the known risk factors were to be
confirmed, no further study would be needed. While this
is on the one hand logical, it also seems superfluous since
the demography of Long Island already is known to include a high percentage of women who fit the high-risk
categories. A further study would only confirm the association.

The only purpose such a study could serve would be
to provide a possible cause other than groundwater. As
Dr. Niebling pointed out, "we do not want our residents
to panic."

Panic, of course, would not be useful in any community, but panic is not something to which the average
community is naturally disposed. It would not cause
panic, for example, if each citizen knew the source of
his or her water supply and its quality—bacterial and
chemical.

In fact, in the face of the potentially distressing news
about the extent of toxic waste and other environmental
contamination and the appearance here and there of
mysterious clusters that science cannot explain, the cit-

izen's only protection is information. For information and knowledge are, naturally, defenses.

Knowing something is generally better than being suspicious about it; information and knowledge can mitigate panic. And as the pattern of leukemia clusters seems to demonstrate, the more ordinary individuals ask, the more scientists tend to learn.

The mirror that the Woburn events held up to environmental epidemiology has made some difference, at least on the question of how far a cluster investigation can go. For example, Woburn surely had to do with the fact that a leukemia cluster investigation in Fairhaven, Massachusetts, was taken one step further than might otherwise have occurred. There, too, was an interesting convergence of circumstances.

Fairhaven, near the shipping center and once-bustling harbor of New Bedford, has roughly 16,000 people. In 1982 a statistically significant cluster of seven cases of leukemia in children under fifteen years of age was confirmed by the CDC after a parent had brought it to official attention. The case control study turned up no common factor and no common history, other than that all the children lived on streets adjacent to Cushman Park, where local children played, and four of the cases actually lived on the border of the park.

New Bedford Harbor had been put on the Superfund priority cleanup list because the harbor sediment was heavily contaminated with polychlorinated biphenyls (PCBs), extremely toxic, non-biodegradable chemicals strongly associated with cancers of various types in laboratory animals.

Harbor dredge had been used to fill in the swampy

area where Cushman Park was created. Initial tests of park soil did not turn up any PCB contamination, but tests of ambient air picked up some levels that were, according to an EPA spokesman, "within the range of national values," although higher than those found at a background station at Darmouth, Massachusetts, a location upwind from New Bedford Harbor. Fairhaven residents had even asked the EPA to look into the piping that ran under the park up from the harbor, on the chance that PCBs infiltrated through that route. It made sense because about the only good thing to say about PCBs from a point of view of environmental testing is that, if they are there, they can usually be found. They are not soluble in water and are very long-lived.

So PCBs were effectively ruled out as a cause of the leukemia cluster in Fairhaven. However, the search for the PCBs did have the effect of stimulating health officials to consider other causes. The New Bedford area was a center of polluting industries that dumped heavy metals, dyes, and a lot of volatile organic contaminants in the harbor at one time or another, most of which can no longer be found.

As John Cutler, the CDC epidemiologist who was sent to investigate Woburn in 1980 and then permanently reassigned to Massachusetts, points out, "do you go on a wild goose chase and sample everything with the hope of coming up with some potential exposure? You could spend a lot of money and generate a very little bit of learning. If you do, it becomes a value judgment." Or a political judgment based on the allocation of resources.

The MDPH, according to Cutler, was "finally funded" to conduct a study to see if something other than PCBs could be found. Even though PCBs cannot be linked to the leukemia cluster, the cluster has stimulated an investigation to determine to what extent the pollution in New Bedford Harbor has infiltrated the bodies of residents in the greater New Bedford area.

Such a study would yield interesting data about how far contaminants travel and how intensely they concentrate in human cells. In the first phase the study would randomly sample 1,400 residents for traces of heavy metals—mercury and cadmium, for example—in their blood. Then if there appears to be a worrying trend, a further "cut" of the data will be made, and those residents who have high levels of heavy metals will also have their blood screened for PCBs and matched with controls for a battery of tests including examination of the immunological system, neurological damage, and liver function—exactly the same sorts of tests done in the Woburn legal case, the Velsicol legal case, and other litigations where "footprints in the snow" are needed for evidence.

The New Bedford study held the promise of showing that a state health monitoring agency can indeed take its classic epidemiological approach further than usual.

That may have some implications for Peabody, Massachusetts, Bruce Young's home town, which is also in the MDPH bailiwick. Like Woburn, it has a long tannery history. Peabody even has its own odor, which wafts around town, especially in summer, emanating from the tanneries still in operation. Peabody too had a statistically significant cluster of deaths from pancreatic cancer. The MDPH, using students from Boston College trained by the department, conducted a questionnaire survey of the cluster families and found no common factor among the victims, nor could it find any correlation with tannery waste sites. As of spring 1985 the investigation had stopped there.

"What we need," said Cutler, "is environmental data that goes back thirty or forty years, and it doesn't exist."

Elaine Krueger of the MDPH, who has also worked at Woburn, New Bedford, and Peabody said, "the lack of biological and environmental data has always been our stumbling block in epidemiology. We have got to find ways of working closer with those who are collecting the basic science or we will never understand any of this."

Of course, there is a danger in moving too fast on the new epidemiological front. Robert Hoover, who has been head of Environmental Epidemiology at the National Cancer Institute since 1972, seemed mindful of the frustration. He said, "there has to be a way to screen out real effects from the ones that are not worth following any further. But we have no systematic way yet to do that."

He believes biochemical epidemiology, or molecular epidemiology, could go "a long way to resolve one of the big concerns," that is, how to prove that ill people have actually suffered an exposure that might damage their body—either to DNA, the immune system, or any of the other body mechanisms whose roles in the preservation of health are only beginning to be examined.

These methods, Hoover admits, "could lead us to a real understanding of how any exposure gets to be a disease." But he also takes a cautious view of the use of innovative theories too early. "This is a science at the very frontier of the laboratory. There is a danger in going too fast. . . . There is a big difference between plodding and exaggerating."

Hoover's fear is not unfounded. There is indeed a danger that molecular epidemiologists, intoxicated by the dazzling array of their refined techniques, may fail to distinguish a finding from a meaning. Says Hoover, "if you have a very sensitive laboratory method that does not find what you suspected was there, you might exonerate a substance that was in fact guilty even though you didn't find it. And by the same token, just because your method was so impressive, you might cling to a notion and assume you are right when you are not."

It is ironic that cluster investigation could be hampered eventually by too much know-how, and studies might be termed "inconclusive" precisely because so many small amounts of different exposures were found that it will be impossible to tell one potential culprit from the other. The difference will be made, as always, by the motives and the quality of the investigations, and by the care with which one foot is put in front of the other.

The meaningful science will come, as Hoover acknowledges, from the scientist who really wants to find a useful answer. By their nature, cluster investigations have been treated as public relations brush fires that had to be put out, with little real planning for what might be learned from them. As Hoover says, "When one of these comes up, most serious investigators are immersed in other work. Digging into a provocative cluster means dropping what you are doing. It means answering the question, is there something that I can do that would advance our knowledge, and making a decision to switch research tracks long enough and far enough to find something. To find funding and so forth gets to be a major undertaking and a very individual thing."

It is not as though the myriad problems of conducting meaningful scientific research on mysterious health patterns did not occur to those who, in recognizing the scope of the toxic waste problem, established the Superfund back in 1980. At that time, when the legislation passed, Congress included a provision that called for the establishment of a new health agency, within the cabinet-level Department of Health and Human Services (HHS), whose task would have been precisely to figure out a way to look for patterns of disease possibly related to toxic waste sites before those patterns came looking for the health agency. In other words, the intent of the Congress, on behalf of the citizenry, and the legislation was to try to eliminate the catch-22, as well as to take full advantage of the latest environmental epidemiology laboratory techniques.

Among other recommendations, Congress mandated that the new health agency conduct surveys, laboratory projects, and chemical testing specifically intended to determine relationships between exposure to toxic substances and illness. Congress also designated the EPA to be the lead agency to administer the Superfund, and the HHS then designated the CDC to carry out the health provisions of the law, by creating a special CDC-Superfund office, rather than an entirely new agency.

Since CDC has traditionally been the nation's most important epidemiological agency, it was sensible to designate the CDC as the spearhead for investigations of what seemed to have the potential to be a new epidemic.

However, four years after the establishment of Superfund, not a single health study had been completed by the CDC-Superfund agency, and very few had begun, according to a report on the agency's activities conducted by the comptroller general of the United States and published in October 1984. And though the scientific impediments to such studies can be formidable, the failure of the CDC to accomplish almost anything related to Superfund was described by the report as strictly due to institutional limitations—bad communication between the EPA and the CDC, budget reductions, and other administrative delays.

One of the major delays took place in 1981, the first year of office for the embattled former EPA director, Anne Gorsuch. According to the comptroller general's report, "EPA impeded HHS' implementation of the law by attempting to limit the department's designated Superfund responsibilities." This impeding took several forms, not the least of which was the outright deletion of all references to HHS's health responsibilities in one of the earliest drafts of how the provisions of Superfund would actually be put into practice. Also because, according to the comptroller's report, "from the start EPA's administrator and assistant administrator for solid waste and emergency response had little interest in cooperating with HHS to implement Superfund activities." The EPA did not make a list of which sites were being designated as priorities to the HHS, despite a request to do so. According to the comptroller's report, "as a result the first 115 priority hazardous waste sites were unknown to the HHS until EPA made the list public in October 1981." The practical effect of this delay was that those who needed to plan where to do health studies had no idea throughout 1981 where they should do health studies first.

There were other clear examples of failure to adhere to the spirit and the letter of Superfund. According to the comptroller general's report, "in another example of EPA attempting to minimize HHS' Superfund role, EPA hired a toxicologist to render health and medical determination regarding Superfund sites, even though health activities had been delegated to HHS. . . . For example, at Ft. Smith, Arkansas, EPA regional officials and Arkansas state health officials agreed that toxic substances posed an immediate public health threat. The EPA toxicologist advised that an immediate public health threat did not exist; therefore, EPA did not believe it was necessary to quickly initiate cleanup activities. Rather than waiting for the EPA to act, the state cleaned up the site on its own."

According to the report the blocks to communication were at the executive level: "the agencies had a good working relationship at the staff level, but when HHS' proposals and projects were forwarded for approval of EPA top managers, they were usually rejected or ignored."

There was also the practical matter of money. For fiscal year 1982 the HHS submitted a budget to the EPA for Superfund-related health studies of $10 million. Of this the EPA, under Anne Gorsuch, and the Office of Management and Budget, under David Stockman, approved $3.3 million. But then, according to the comptroller general's report, it took five months for the two agencies to sign a formal "interagency agreement" so that the funds could literally be transferred to the HHS, with the result that, absent the agreement, "HHS was able to accomplish little under Superfund except to organize its coordinating group, because no staff or funds were available for the health-related activities specified in the approved budget."

Congress, in an attempt to increase the money available to HHS, directed the EPA to make an additional $3.7 million available to the HHS. The money was appropriated, but HHS never requested it. Consequently, because of failure to hire staff and to literally take the money out of the bank, as of September 8, 1982, about $5.9 million remained unused by HHS for its Superfund-related activities.

In 1983, still failing to use the funds to its credit, HHS requested a $21 million appropriation. It received $3.2 million. In 1984 HHS requested $6.4 million; the Office of Management and Budget cut the item to $1.9 million. Congress restored the appropriation to $5 million. This brought the total amount of money available to the HHS to $16.9 million, of which during the first six months of the 1984 fiscal year, HHS had spent $3.5 million.

In short, according to the comptroller general's report, because of bureaucratic delay, indifference to the priority of health studies by key executive personnel who set up the Superfund, and lack of initiative, the health agency assigned the task of assessing the health effects of toxic waste sites had, four years after its job had been defined, made practically no progress.

The comptroller general's report concluded that the "working relationship" between the EPA and the HHS had improved, and it suggested that in 1985 the delayed health projects could begin. But even these would not necessarily yield much fruit, given the amount of time that elapsed since their conception.

As of 1985 the health studies on the CDC docket were based on an EPA determination of which sites were the most likely to be causing health effects, given the toxic properties of the substances found at the waste site, their quantities, and their mix.

Several sites selected for study were chosen because they contained the highly toxic dioxin.

The CDC also planned to study the effects of arsenic on the population that lived near a copper smelter in Ruston, Washington, which shut down in March of 1985. Several years prior, when the smelter was operating, children in the area were found to have high concentrations of arsenic in their hair and urine. These data were collected in connection with standards for arsenic exposure that the EPA was attempting to set for smelters that produced exceptionally high arsenic emissions. The HHS would presumably be able to collect information that can be compared to that which was collected earlier, and this may indeed yield useful information on the effects of arsenic in the body. However, in terms of protecting a population from ongoing danger, the study was rendered basically moot by the closure of the smelter, and any carcinogenic potential would have already been set in motion.

Delay, as noted in the New Brighton, Minnesota, case, can be especially damaging to studies of effects of contaminated groundwater and health. And perhaps the most dramatic example involves the Verona well field in Battle Creek, Michigan, a location where, as of April 1985, the CDC-Superfund office was about to begin an investigation.

In 1981, while Calhoun County, Michigan, officials were investigating a chemical spill on the site of a small company, they sampled the water in the company's wells. When they found the water contained solvents, the officials informed the company that the spill seemed to have contaminated their private wells. The company, however, informed the agency that it used only municipal water.

Further checks of some thirty municipal wells found twenty-eight to be contaminated, some with no less than sixty different chemical substances. About 100 residential homes that had private wells were also affected, the highest level of contamination climbing to 4,000 ppb. Ultimate investigations found that the chemical plume, which had already traveled a full mile, had originated with several solvent and waste hauling companies whose underground holding tanks were found to be leaking extensively. The state of Michigan eventually prosecuted the dumpers, who were found guilty, but one of the largest contaminators ultimately filed bankruptcy, and so it was difficult to recover any cleanup costs.

And according to Ruffin Harris, executive director of the Hazardous Waste Organizing Alliance, a nonprofit group that works with communities affected by toxic waste contamination, Michigan officials were extremely reluctant to call any attention to the problem of the Battle Creek water because several large employers, namely the leading companies in the breakfast cereal industry, had also been using the contaminated water. This raised the specter that cereal cooked using the water was also contaminated, although the companies said that their processes would have eliminated such a possibility because cooking would "strip" off the chemicals and vent them into the manufacturing plant. Though this might have posed a risk to the workers in the plant, presumably venting did not pose a threat to all the boxes of cereal on shelves around America.

In the meantime, no alternative sources of water were made available to residents who had received a letter advising them not to use their wells. They were told that they could pick up "clean" water at a municipal pumping station, but no bottled water or emergency shower facilities near the residences were provided. According to Harris, it was only a sit-in by residents carried out at the governor of Michigan's office in 1982 that led to the provision of bottled water. Residents also told the governor of the concern for their health, and the governor, newly elected, made a public commitment to a health study.

According to Harris a questionnaire prepared by the CDC was circulated and critiqued by residents and discussed with state health officials. Ruffin says it was eventually withdrawn, and he was told that it was being redrafted. In the fall of 1983 the residents and the Hazardous Waste Organizing Alliance undertook their own health study. Blood samples were collected from eleven residents and screened for liver damage. According to Harris, only one of the eleven subjects had liver enzyme readings within the normal range.

Half the population depending on contaminated well

water are children, and the neighborhood is composed of generally low-income white families whose houses might be worth roughly $10,000 if the water had not been contaminated.

As of April 1985 the community had not been informed when the CDC was actually going to begin its work. And though the residents were the only ones who had collected any biological samples in the matter, no public health official requested a copy of the results or to speak with the medical personnel who had taken the tests. Two new wells had been dug by the EPA, but according to Harris, because of financial considerations they were dug on land the city already owned, and therefore they were in the path of the traveling contaminating plume.

About the most interesting projects under way at the CDC relating to detecting health clusters involves the Sentinel Surveillance System, which was in the planning stages in the spring of 1985, having been funded for the first year for $250,000. The idea had been proposed within CDC, according to Dr. Matthew Zack, several years ago, but funding for it was first made available in fiscal year 1984.

Though Dr. Zack and Dr. Glyn Caldwell devised the program within the CDC, the concept of sentinel diseases derives, according to Zack, from studies done by Dr. David D. Rutstein at the Harvard School of Public Health. A sentinel surveillance system works in keeping with its name. Its intent is to look for disease patterns and perhaps intervene in time, if not to stop the exposure, to learn something from the pattern.

The sentinel disease concept aims to discover what

about a disease could have been prevented. Tracing each case of the disease thoroughly, medicine can discover what about it might have been preventable. By eliminating one by one the preventable components, the disease itself could ultimately be eliminated.

The clearest example of this approach was seen in the 1930s in the decline in the number of deaths of women during pregnancy and childbirth. At that time in the United States, when such deaths were not uncommon, many hospitals in the country had maternal mortality boards, whose sole purpose was to look into every maternal death in the hospital. These investigations turned up practices that could be changed—nutritional factors, antiseptic factors, aspects related to prenatal care. Thus maternal death became an essentially preventable disease.

The sentinel system has other parallels. It is the approach taken by epidemiologists in search of infectious epidemics. When reports of such diseases as measles or polio came into the CDC, each and every case was investigated, regardless of how many there were or where they occurred. Today, one case of polio in the United States warrants the level of investigation reserved for epidemics.

The National Institute of Occupational Safety and Health (NIOSH) also worked with the concept of sentinel disease to identify illnesses in workplaces. A sentinel system whose universe began outside the workplace would amount to the first real chance to find clusters that could be caused by environmental contaminants before they find epidemiologists.

According to Zack, the CDC system would look at

sentinel diseases for which several specific causes are already known. These would include rare cancers like angiosarcoma, closely associated with exposure to vinyl chloride, and mesothelioma, closely associated with exposure to asbestos. The system, however, would also look at other diseases known to be sometimes caused by environmental exposures, such as aplastic anemia, which can be caused by exposure to powerful chemicals such as benzene, or as the case of Jimmy Anderson demonstrates, powerful chemical medications.

A sentinel surveillance system would "kick out" every case, for example, of aplastic anemia in the area the system covered, regardless of specific location, say every case within a state regardless of town, and most importantly, regardless of whether the overall incidence was considered "abnormal." The very existence of one case of the disease would be considered abnormal enough to come to the CDC's attention.

Then the sentinel investigating team, much like detectives, would comb the records of the case to see if any of the known causative agents are present in the history of the patient. If so, in theory that causative agent could be investigated and taken out of circulation. If there are none of the known causes—say an angiosarcoma in connection with exposure to a chemical never before associated with the disease—then the CDC might have a framework in which to isolate previously unknown causative factors. A sentinel case would be correlated too for its proximity and potential exposure to toxic waste dumps.

Such a system would pick up a "cluster" that was not in the same town, it would be able to account for the latency factor, and it could generate a lot of useful data about the causes of diseases. It would also avoid many of the problems of "statistical power," because it would not be concerned at first with how many cases of a disease there are. Thus its business would not be verifying clusters, but discovering them. Also, at some point it would be necessary to see whether factors in common among the cases were coincidental. But says Zack, "we might get some false positives, but at least we will not be spending a lot of time and money on an in-depth case control study which might also give false positives."

From the point of view of public health the sentinel has the potential to prevent disease and clusters because one case will be enough to catch public attention, and, for example, a developing cluster of angiosarcomas could be nipped in the bud if the source of vinyl chloride exposure were found before the number of diagnoses had piled high enough to capture attention. Of course, because of the long latency factor for some cancers, a sentinel system will be useless in preventing the first cases to appear in its system. The promise is that it might prevent other ones. And even more, a sentinel system could prevent serious diseases, such as anemias, or birth defects, whose environmental causes might well otherwise go entirely unnoticed.

With the initial $250,000 Zack will be at work determining how to adapt current disease registries to the sentinel idea. Ultimately some birth defects will also be added to the sentinel system. Assuming there is a practical way of picking up sentinel diseases fast enough after they occur to make an investigation of them feasible, the sentinel system might be making its first investigations and have some results by the late 1980s. In its first years, Dr. Zack and colleagues, sitting at computer terminals in cramped offices in barrack-style buildings, will amount to the nation's most meaningful surveillance system for toxic waste–related illness.

Ironically, what the sentinel system does is put together the earliest ideas of epidemiology—the epidemiology of the mosquito and malaria—with the complexities of modern environmental contamination. It is a basic idea that could have been implemented sooner. Zack, who seemed hopeful about the possibilities of the sentinel system, said, "it really is just a matter of bringing things together. There is nothing new under the sun in this." And clearly, the system's ultimate success will depend on the financial resources and the human energies appropriated to it. And at this level—the level of concrete commitment—was where national politics nettled the workings of the HHS, the EPA, and Superfund in the first place.

For the matter of what national resources will be allocated to resolving issues of health, toxic waste, and environmental protection does tend to be reduced to politics. Events like the leukemia cluster at Woburn can stimulate political thinking on every governmental level up from the local city hall. But the politics that set the tone are national.

19

The Politics of Science

THE ESTIMATE by epidemiologists Doll and Peto that less than 8% of all cancers are probably caused by pollution, food additives, and occupation or industrial products is the lowest reading available on the number of cancers caused by substances to which individuals are involuntarily exposed. In that there are approximately 870,000 new cancer cases diagnosed each year in the United States, the 8% estimate means that roughly 53,000 cancer cases are preventable in the sense that removal of the carcinogens would prevent the cancers from occurring.

But removing carcinogens requires regulatory action, which, because it affects both the economy of the society and the health of the people in it, becomes political.

And in the mid-1980s the political dimensions of environmental regulation have intensified.

In 1984 a book entitled *The Apocalyptics: Cancer and the Big Lie* was published, and its dust jacket said it revealed the "most astonishing scientific scandals of our time: the ideological corruption of cancer research in the U.S.," which had been "saturating the U.S. with theories of cancer that are pure myth." The book is extremely carefully written, and it takes apart virtually every study ever produced in the United States that found associations between a particular carcinogen and an industrial process. In addition, the book dismisses the idea that tests done on animals can possibly have any relevance for man and concludes that the most serious carcinogens are "natural," that is, found in nature, and are not the by-products of an industrial society. Carcinogens in the "natural" category included asbestos, arsenic, chromium, and tobacco. Lemons, the author pointed out, contains chemicals that could be considered carcinogenic. Even oxygen, perhaps the most essential element on earth, was put in the category of natural carcinogens. It is true that singlet oxygen, a highly reactive form of oxygen that accounts for less than 1% of all natural oxygen, can be dangerous, but the author does not make the distinction, saying instead "man has only the choice to die immediately without oxygen or to die of it eventually."

The author's basic contention is that the "environmental movement," beginning with the writings of Rachel Carson, had American industry as its target and that scientists, particularly epidemiologists who worked for government agencies such as the National Cancer Institute and the Occupational Safety and Health Administration, had been lassoed into the conspiracy. The book suggests, "Epidemiologists, like animal and bacterial extrapolators, are deeply politicized; all are perfectly well aware of the practical implications of their various estimates, and all are perfectly aware that what they are fighting over is the body of industrial civilization."

The book points out that many studies which purport

to link industrial pollutants and toxic waste products to cancer have been discredited for sloppiness and unfounded premises and implies that it was a desire to impugn the reputation of the economic system of the country that fed this poor professional approach. In fact, after a lecture about her book the author gave at New York University in January 1985, the implication was made more explicit. While smoking a cigarette and answering a question about what she thought the ultimate underlying motive for the poor science had been, she said, "I think it came out of a leftist movement in science."

One of the studies the author gave most credibility was the 1981 report by Doll and Peto in which they did indeed criticize a number of studies which they believed had made statements about the extent of environmentally induced cancer on the basis of too scant data. However, Doll and Peto made other statements that were not emphasized in the *The Apocalyptics*.

For example, as to why they had estimated the environmental causes at less than 8%, Doll and Peto said, "our estimate of the small proportions of current cancer mortality due to occupation, pollution, etc. relate, of course, chiefly to those factors for which it has been possible to secure some direct evidence of an effect on humans. Many substances have begun to be used in recent years that are mutagenic to bacteria and carcinogenic in one or more species of laboratory animals. How far exposure to these substances will contribute to the production of cancer in humans in the future is a matter for speculation. On general biological principles . . . it must be assumed that some (though not all) of these substances will involve a risk of cancer and, even though the doses to which humans are exposed are commonly minute in comparison with those used in laboratory experiments, this is not always the case and some harmful effects must be anticipated."

Doll and Peto also said about studies that do not pick up evidence of health effects, "negative human evidence may mean very little unless it relates to prolonged and heavy exposure." And of their attributing a fraction of environmentally induced cancer to industrial products, they said, "Although we can attribute a nominal 'less than 1%' . . . to such products, we must reiterate our conclusion from some previous sections: There is too much ignorance for complacency to be justified."

And as for what action to take, Doll and Peto said, "the intelligent use of laboratory tests should provide a powerful means for the prevention of new hazards in the future. It will, however, be difficult to use them confidently until we have more exact knowledge of the mechanisms of human carcinogenesis and of the various different classes of factors that can accelerate or retard these mechanisms. . . . The use of particular tests to establish approximate priorities for action on the few agents which by that test seem most dangerous may already be practicable."

If it is scientifically reasonable to anticipate future hazards, then government would apparently have a responsibility to regulate hazards on the basis of prudence. Human beings should not be involuntarily exposed to substances that are reasonably likely to be dangerous. True, regulatory policy is in a bind when there is little data on which to base conclusions, but prudent government can reasonably regulate on the basis of what is known already and on what can be hypothetically surmised.

And in March 1985, leaders of major chemical companies testified at congressional hearings that they would support, in fact welcome, new federal government standards controlling hazardous airborne emissions. Harold J. Corbett, senior vice-president of the Monsanto Company, which once owned chemical operations in Woburn, said the industry's position came from their recognition that the public "simply does not have faith that the chemical industry will regulate itself in the public interest." And if there are regulations in place to which companies adhere, and accidents still occur, companies would be more likely to be able to sustain claims with their own insurance companies for leaks and spills than they can without stiff regulation.

But in the mid-1980s the administration of the federal government was elected for a second term on the theme that government regulation was something to be lessened, not enhanced. Interestingly, as political vapors rose that tended to diminish the importance of regulation, increased public policy emphasis was put on "lifestyle factors" in cancer causation, such as diet, smoking, and alcohol consumption, those variables one voluntarily introduces in one's life. Sometimes this is simplistically called the "blame-the-victim" approach to cancer causation, but it does tend to put the major responsibility on the individual for avoiding cancer rather than on the government for eliminating carcinogenic substances from the environment.

In 1982 the American Cancer Society began a survey

of 1.2 million Americans, to cost approximately $12 million, chiefly to determine individually avoidable factors in life-style—eating of spicy foods, use of mouthwash, and so forth—that might be correlated with a pattern of cancer mortality. Also, the American Cancer Society published a diet that recommended individuals lower their consumption of fatty foods and eat more whole grains to reduce the risk of cancer. And when in March of 1985 the president of the United States was found to have a polyp in his intestines, the White House announced widely that the president had been placed on the society's "anticancer" diet to ensure the benign polyp did not become malignant, thus sending the message to the American people that cancer prevention was as simple as changing the food on the table.

Certainly dietary factors, mostly nutritional, according to Doll and Peto, play a role in the development of cancer, and certainly the public may weary of the drumbeat of news that this or that substance has been found to be carcinogenic. Even Dr. Joseph Fraumeni, chief of the Environmental Epidemiology Branch of the National Cancer Institute, who was widely criticized in *The Apocalyptics* for being alarmist about the role of occupational and industrial causes of cancer, noted during an interview in his Bethesda, Maryland, office that dietary and other factors are quite important and that it was incorrect for the public to perceive science as generating fear of the "carcinogen of the week."

But exaggeration can only inevitably brew from an informational and administrative process that includes miscommunication of complicated scientific results by scientists and their "roaring" at each other, the cycle of

denial by anyone who has a stake in the continued production or sale of any substance accused of being carcinogenic or implicated in a health problem such as
Woburn's, media "hype," and the inherent limitations
of the epidemiological study methods. So while it is
irresponsible to fan public concern over nothing, it is
equally irresponsible to give the public the impression
that prudent regulation is a burden that should be shak-
en off as soon as possible.

For a drop in public esteem for prudent regulation
will coincide with a rise in technology's ability to detect contamination. Increasingly sharp measuring techniques now find contamination in the parts per billion
range, and if public officials or industry representatives
belittle these findings, what can the average person be
left to think? If the public comes to believe that locating
environmental contamination is merely a matter of
"seek and ye shall find" because scientific tools are over-
ly sensitive or because scientists who "find things" have
spurious intentions, it would seem that the entire system
for controlling environmental health hazards would suffer a widespread perhaps irreversible crumbling of credibility.

The attitude that government regulation is a burden
filters down to local officials. They transfer their ani-
mosity to the body of authority most closely regulating
them—usually the state government. And if these local
officials are skeptical of the overall merit of environmental regulation, they easily can transmit a sense of
indifference to environmental threats that may be
brought to their attention by the people of their town
or area. And local officials are likely to be the first level

of government that must respond to the discovery of local environmental problems, such as possible clusters.

In Woburn, for example, the skepticism of the value of regulations among some local officials can sometimes be clear. The city engineer, an affable man who was at the center of the maelstrom over wells G and H, said "the state . . . they are always in your pocket with some other thing they want you to do." The city public works commissioner, while on one hand respecting the state of Massachusetts for wanting to protect public water supplies, also had no real appetite for learning what the DEQE had found in its samples of Horn Pond water after the sludge chambers were found in the swimming pool excavation in 1984. Though he carefully pointed out how important the Horn Pond aquifer was to Woburn's water supply, when asked what was found there, he simply said, "I don't know. The state is taking care of that. You have to ask them what they found."

At more or less the same time as the White House announced the president's adoption of the anticancer diet, it also announced his plan for a $5.3 billion appropriation for the reauthorization of Superfund. The plan did not include a provision to compensate victims. And it sought to restrict use of Superfund funds strictly to cleanup of the dumps per se. Under this plan the funding that permitted study of the groundwater flow in Woburn, New Brighton, and various other places would be eliminated. In other words, funds for determining who caused contamination of groundwater were deleted from the administration's plan.

The plan also transferred the bulk of the government's share of cleanup costs from the federal government to state governments on the theory that they had budget surpluses which could generate the funds. Taxes on waste haulers and chemical producers would also pay a share of the cleanup costs, and Lee Thomas, the head of the EPA, said that interest earned on "unused Superfund money" and court settlements on enforcement cases brought by the EPA would complete the Superfund financial package.

Though the president's statement said his recommendations for the Superfund program would "allow us to move aggressively forward to eliminate the health and environmental risks associated with past waste disposal practices," according to Congressman James Florio of New Jersey, the structure of the plan actually meant that it would take approximately thirty years to clean up the priority waste sites.

And the elimination of funds to do physical research at the sites on the extent of contamination of water and air effectively meant that specific health effects, which might come to light as clusters, could not be adequately investigated because no data could be generated— except by private institutions—that could be used to link cause to effect.

The president's approach to Superfund, then, would have further institutionalized the frustrating limits of science exemplified by the Woburn events. And outside of Superfund there were no other public programs in place or planned that could begin to effectively break this cycle. As of 1985 the only way for the Woburn events to be discovered would be exactly the way they were discovered before—by observant individuals gathering their own data and putting them on the table of those in a position to analyze them.

The failure to look ahead in matters of how to tell

chance occurrences from real ones is not just a failure
of administrative responsibility. It is a failure of thinking, a failure to look at a linear problem in a nonlinear
way. Instead the management of the most best-known
toxic waste problems is rife with questionable solutions
that fail to take long-term impact on individuals into
account.

At Love Canal, for example, in early 1985, as part of
a plan to reclaim the area for habitable living, the re-
clamation agency proposed to issue a clear map that
would indicate to those who might be considering moving into the area which homes had been contaminated
and which had not and to board up the "bad houses"
and encourage sale of the good.

As Dr. Martha Fowlkes, a professor of sociology at
Smith College who studied the Love Canal situation extensively, wondered, "Had no one considered the actual
practical effect on people of dividing the street where
they lived into poisoned and unpoisoned? Who should
be expected to live in an area spotted with stigmatized
houses? Who would want to? It was a program for the
creation of a slum into which the government was asking
others to move. Choosing which so-called habitable
house to buy next to which uninhabitable one is not
having much to choose from."

Indeed the problems of environmental contamination often pose options to citizens that offer little real
choice. Increasingly the tendency to compare the health
benefit of certain health regulations to their economic
costs puts the public in an extremely difficult position.

Such was the case at the ASARCO smelter in Ruston,
Washington, near Tacoma, which was emitting sulfur

dioxide, an odorless gas and known irritant of the respiratory system, associated with emphysema, bronchitis, and other lung ailments; and arsenic, the toxic, tasteless substance believed to have been the poison that killed Napoleon, also strongly associated with human lung and skin cancer. When it became clear that because of depressed prices in the copper industry, ASARCO might shut the smelter down rather than install the equipment necessary to reduce the emissions, William Ruckelshaus, as head of EPA, held hearings intended to ask residents whether they could accept the risk of living in the vicinity of a copper smelter that emitted substances known to be hazardous to human health.

Complying with the sulfur dioxide emissions standards would have meant an investment of $150 million and an unknown amount to meet the arsenic standard, which had yet to be set. Federal EPA experts concluded that arsenic emissions at the Ruston smelter probably caused four lung cancer cases a year in the area and that state-of-the-art technology could reduce the risk to two per year. ASARCO disputed the assessments.

So the public was tossed the question of what is a job worth compared to the risk of cancer. Two cases, four—how many is too many, and who is to say? This type of public involvement has spawned a new science in itself, "risk management," which in complicated situations can be used by those whose task it is to make tough decisions to avoid the decision. As William Ruckelshaus said, "For me to sit here in Washington and tell the people of Tacoma what is an acceptable risk would be at best arrogant and at worst inexcusable."

At the risk hearings Ruckelshaus called, residents of

the area wore lapel buttons that said "BOTH," meaning both jobs and a safe environment. Most of the residents testifying indicated that they would accept some risk— they could not be guaranteed no risk at all—if the company installed the state-of-the-art technology available in order to retain the jobs the smelter provided. But ASARCO nevertheless spent $60 million to shut the smelter down, thus eliminating 500 jobs for residents and $32 million in annual tax revenue for the state of Washington. "BOTH," the shutdown said, was something the people could not have.

William Ruckelshaus left the EPA in 1984, but his replacement at the helm, Lee Thomas, who used to head the hazardous waste program, also said he believes strongly in involving the public in risk policy decisions. Also, for example, the appointment in the fall of 1984 of Christopher J. Daggett to head the northeast region of EPA, which takes in Love Canal, further highlighted the emphasis on public involvement. Daggett gave a talk entitled "Risk: A Matter of Education" at a major environmental conference in Rochester, New York, shortly after his appointment that tended to equate public information with public relations. He said, "A major goal of today's EPA is education . . . to put the public's fear to rest about all things chemical . . . a safe world cannot be a zero risk world, and the only way out of this quandary is to let the public take part in the process of evaluating the risks and the benefits."

However, trading off the complexities of the science involved in thoughtfully evaluating future risk with the here-and-now concrete reality of a job and a paycheck puts the individual in an almost untenable situation.

Many would choose a job over the undefined prospect of cancer. And though it is important for the public to know the scientific complexities involved and give them some thought, one wonders if it is not an abrogation of government responsibility to offer its citizens a lesser of two evils choice, particularly when matters of health and diseases like cancer are at stake.

In problems of the complexity of how to unravel and deal with problems caused by environmental pollution in general and toxic waste contamination of resources in particular, indeed it is the quality of leadership, the quality of the thinking brought to bear on the problem, that can inspire good solutions or hammer out duds.

For as Dr. Fowlkes and a Smith College colleague, Dr. Patricia Miller, pointed out in a paper presented at the annual meetings of the American Sociological Association in August 1985, increasing technological advance can present unprecedented challenges to both leaders and citizens. Technology not only creates the potential for acute accidents such as the leak of lethal gas in Bhopal, India, in December 1984 that killed more than 2,000 people but also the possibility of what the authors call "unnatural disasters": nonacute events that involve "uncontrolled exposure to invisible environmental contaminants with an unbounded potential for risk." Unnatural disasters are "gratuitous events, originating in the application of technology in the face of risk which is paradoxically both certain and uncertain."

In an unnatural disaster a few leitmotifs appear. For one the risk in question usually becomes publicly known long after it is suspected or recognized by an individual behind the scenes. For example, officials in Hooker

Chemical Company knew that land they were offering the school board for a playground was soaked with chemicals, but it did not point that out to the school board. For their part, school board officials knew that to secure the lease for the land, they had to indemnify Hooker against liability but did not ask what it was Hooker wanted to be indemnified against.

Also, in an unnatural disaster, events do not happen in a flash; they unfold. The passage of time, according to Fowlkes and Miller, acts as a "cultural medium transforming and modifying the original circumstances in ways that render the relationship between cause and effect highly obscure, even to the extent of casting doubt on whether either a 'cause' or an 'effect' actually exists." For example, at Woburn, though Anne Anderson had the feeling that the leukemia cases were clumping in time as well as place, had the diagnoses come on fast and furiously, one a month, for example, the fact that a cluster existed might have been officially recognized sooner.

Too, unnatural disasters impose a definition of "normal" on those who perceive the unfolding events as abnormal. Anne Anderson, in fact, was in constant inner turmoil about whether she was right or paranoid. In fact the battle ultimately joined by Bruce Young was at first one simply to establish that an abnormal situation truly existed.

Unnatural disasters are generally wrapped in scientific ambiguity, and the ambiguity, according to Fowlkes and Miller, is "likely to be exploited on behalf of whatever competing interests are involved." But perhaps the most important dimension of the unnatural disaster is aptly demonstrated by Woburn—the fact that

victims are difficult to identify by conventional defini-
tions. Consequently, if there are no victims to be found,
then there can have been no disaster. Fowlkes and Miller
conclude, "The most insidious feature of the unnatural
disaster, then, is its capacity to become increasingly
widespread at the same time that it goes unrecognized
and its unidentified casualties increase proportion-
ately."

The absence of appropriate epidemiological methods
to identify causes and effects, the slow-moving cleanup
action at Superfund sites, the tendency to hold regulatory science in low regard, along with the opposite tendency to admire the science that points out the importance of an individual's control on the factors affecting
health, and our inability to discern clusters of ill health
possibly related to toxic waste dumps would seem to
leave us prey to a veritable cornucopia of unnatural
disasters.

If so, at what point does "needing to know" conflict
with not wanting to know, and when does indifference
or incompetence become negligence—if not legal, then
moral? These are questions that the public will have to
ask itself along with how much health risk it regards as
acceptable.

Such difficult questions place serious demands on
individuals to resist the tendency to wish all things were
black or white and especially to resist the politicization
of the science which says that any provocative conclusion is the brainchild of troublemaking, even perhaps
subversive, environmentalist in scientific disguise.

For the tendency to polarize public policy matters
that depend on science tends also to polarize the sci-

entific facts themselves. Thus scientific results are expressed in either-or terms, and science divides into
camps: the genetic theory versus the epigenetic; the theory that it is a "zap" of a carcinogen that causes cancer
versus the idea that a "cascade" of carcinogenic events
are set in motion. The zap and the cascade are not mutually exclusive, but they somehow come across to the
public as separate roads to the same hotel. In truth, they
are intersecting, mutually dependent theories.

The fact is that the history of science is full of either-
or arguments that obscured important truths for a long
time. Ultimately it is people who make the difference
between whether a knotty situation like Woburn gets
properly unraveled or not. Some people directly seek
the truth, while others think of truth as an accidental
by-product of their daily routine. Sometimes the difference is in the individual energies of a particular person.
There are those who when they make a call and hear a
busy signal dial again immediately, and then there are
those who wait so long to place the call again that they
find their party has since gone out. Finding truth is often
a matter of making the opportunity to do so and of not
giving up because the prevailing view is contrary to
what is suggested by the nugget of an idea.

Massachusetts Legislator Nicholas Paleologos observed the Woburn events from a mixed vantage point—
that of a life-long Woburn resident with legitimate concerns for his own health, an elected politician with a
responsibility to all his constituents, whether or not they
were suffering leukemia in their families, and an academic observer of the conduct of public affairs. He
thinks that in matters relating to environmental health

hazards, institutional inertia, except when it comes to saying what has *not* been found, plays a large role in creating crises in community confidence in public health agencies and scientific knowledge in general, and in particular, in the unrolling of events in Woburn.

Close to the political process and the conflict between "old hands" and "new guard," he characterizes governmental apparatuses as replete with shifting interests and shifting emphases on whom it is the government should respond to—the press, the people, itself. Most people, he said, think mostly about what they can do to smooth a problem over, not what they can do to understand it. In these surroundings, he says, "it is a rare individual who becomes consumed with getting to the bottom of a complicated situation. And that is the kind of person that it takes."

And science, on which any ultimate understanding of a cluster like Woburn's must depend, is not immune to these flaws and blockages. The importance of curiosity in any process of discovery makes it difficult to say that science proceeds by rational plan rather than accidental happenings.

What comes first, one might ask, the microscope or the desire to see microbes; the x-ray crystallograph of DNA or the passion to see the structure of the most important molecule in the body; the gas chromatograph mass spectrometer or the wish to know what is in drinking water?

The inherent desire to know can often make the difference between science from which others can learn and science that goes along to get along. Of course, while some individuals are simply not inquisitive and others are outright close-minded, there are also some inherent structural features of the scientific establishment that underline resistance to new ideas. That resistance can often be nonrational, according to Dr. Thomas S. Kuhn, a physicist and philosopher at the Massachusetts Institute of Technology and author of the book *The Structure of Scientific Revolutions.* At a forum held by the *New York Times* in March 1983, he said, "it is not just stubbornness that leads people to hold on to an outmoded belief. This is something built into scientific language and technique."

In other words, the building block nature of science creates "givens" and assumptions on which other scientists proceed. Recognizing a new discovery means assumptions may have to be shed that in some cases have been long held. Often a discovery is made by nothing more complicated than taking a fresh look at an established belief.

Dr. Joshua Lederberg, president of Rockefeller University in New York City, holds his Nobel Prize in biology up as an example. He won the prize for showing in the 1940s, at the age of twenty-one, that bacteria had genetics and sexuality, which widely flouted conventional scientific theory at the time. In fact, Lederberg noted the belief that bacteria did not sexually reproduce had even been enshrined in the scientific classification Schizomycetes, which means "fission fungi." Beings that reproduce by fission, that is, one entity splitting into two, could not be the result of two entities combining into one. At the same *New York Times* forum, he said, "I have felt that the discovery should have been made twenty years before I was born. One can hardly give a rational explanation for the fact that it had not even been looked for."

In fact, according to Kuhn, Lederberg's discovery could only be accepted once several other basic notions changed as well, most fundamentally, the notion that a "pure" bacterial culture was one in which bacteriologists prevented bacteria from undergoing any change. If a bacteriologist at the time saw a change in a culture of bacteria, he or she might assume the culture had been somehow tainted and the experiment spoiled. So, Kuhn pointed out, "That type of assumption made it hard to discover that there are genetically borne changes in bacteria . . . you'd have to change your ideas of the appropriate techniques for purification to accept a discovery of the sort Dr. Lederberg made."

There are some tempting parallels to be made with the way the Harvard biostatistics department study at Woburn was criticized. Before the study's significance could be accepted, epidemiologists would have had to abandon preconceptions of what makes a "pure" study and what are appropriate epidemiological techniques, such as that disease classifications must conform to an accepted nomenclature or that community volunteers must of necessity introduce bias.

Drawing the relationship between common sense and scientific thought, Lederberg pointed out, "To the extent that very little by way of scientific demonstration follows formal procedures, it is pretty much common sense. Scientists use methods we should recognize in daily life but that we may not push to the ultimate. . . . But there's a relentlessness in science rarely found in everyday affairs. Indeed if we did find it, we'd call the person who operated like this compulsive." Unless perhaps that person were a mother whose son had died of leukemia for reasons that could have been prevented. Then that compulsive person might be called "emotionally involved."

The importance of multidisciplined research to scientific advance also seemed self-evident to Lederberg. He believed that had geneticists and bacteriologists "rubbed their noses in each other's work," the discovery he made might have been made sooner. Dr. Kuhn responded that evolutionary patterns and developments internal to science "most fruitfully" bring scientific disciplines together and that the sharing process cannot be sped or rationalized. Lederberg however argued for a more deliberate attempt to put disciplines in touch with each other. He said, as though characterizing the debate over what constitutes appropriate epidemiology in the case of Woburn, "institutional forms have consequences; one can do something about those forms. . . . Permissions for disciplines to meet one another aren't that easy to come by. Many institutional settings would not allow scientists to change the character and direction of an investigation or to enter fields in which they did not have credentials. It would argue that creating environments where these things are permissible, even if you can't force two nuclei to fuse, is an important issue of science management."

In other words, in any branch of science, what one finds is a function of how one looks, how far one takes a question, who one talks to, and who is doing the looking. And it would seem especially clear in the complicated case of environmental epidemiology where study after study seems to meet similar impediments to establishing cause and effect. Indeed, even Doll and Peto, who take a very conservative view of the extent of the role played by environmental contaminants in the cause of cancer, point out the need for a new, more imaginative scientific approach.

While calling for additional classic case-control epidemiological studies on as large a scale as is practicable, they also say, "the one trouble with any such studies is that the questions they answer *are only those already posited.* It may be no bad thing to answer these, but it should be obvious from our review of current lines of research how far current cancer research may be from even knowing the right questions to ask."

In this context, given a full understanding of the complexities involved in environmental health, one knows that despite the best efforts there are questions for which there is legitimately no answer. Yet one must wonder if the prevalence of "inconclusive" studies in environmental epidemiology represents the legitimate limits of rigorous creative thinking or merely an institutionalized, politicized refrain.

20

The Aftermath

A STIFF MORNING BREEZE can roll a basketball from one
yard to the next in East Woburn which, twenty years
after the Andersons moved in, remains primarily a residential neighborhood of newly shingled homes, shaved
log fences, and family dogs resting on asphalt driveways
just wide enough for one car. Sometimes so many children get off the school bus on Orange Street that the
block looks like a playground of children dawdling and
slowly making their way home.

Outside the Anderson house a Sunday morning might
find Chuck Anderson working on the stripped steel
sheath of his car, a large radio echoing its music up
under the chassis while he fiddles with a wire, leaving
only his long legs visible. Inside, his sister Christine,
wrapped in a deep purple shaggy bathrobe, might well
be talking on the telephone with a friend about where
to look for a first apartment away from home. Luciano
Pavarotti, a favorite of Anne Anderson's, might be belt-
ing an aria across the kitchen where Anne herself might
well be reading a newspaper, a cup of steaming coffee
by her side.

There have been many public committees formed
since toxic waste and the contamination of wells G and

H were discovered in Woburn—watchdog committees, legislative advisory committees, health department planning committees, environmental monitoring committees. Anne Anderson is rarely asked to sit on them officially. This could be a legacy from the earliest days of the cluster investigation when she preferred that her name not appear publicly lest the credibility carried by Bruce Young's position as a church pastor be diluted by the involvement of a mother who had so much personally at stake. She says it was only at Bruce Young's urging that she began to feel comfortable with public recognition of her role.

"Maybe people on long-term committees are afraid I'll get hysterical," she says, but adds, in a characteristically calm, measured voice, "I have never been hysterical, just frustrated at times when people tend to forget real children died and real families suffered." She remembers one meeting she did attend where some other members made jokes about the poor drinking water in the conference room and how they might get leukemia if they drank it. When Anne Anderson did not laugh, the others stopped laughing.

Often, however, she is asked to be an "observer" at various official functions related to toxic waste issues, and she gladly does so. She has sat on the sidelines as legislators tried to draft pieces of law that try to describe what makes a "toxic waste victim." She has seen them argue for several hours over whether wording in a sentence is too "jazzy" or too "heavy."

Anne Anderson has worked with For a Clean Environment (FACE) since its inception and was instrumental in the organization's securing several grants from foundations with national recognition. She has spent years of days sitting behind the desk in the Main Street office writing letters, taking calls from other communities around the country seeking advice on how to establish they have a health problem, or answering questions from reporters and public figures about what is new in Woburn. The leukemia cluster and its aftermath consumes most of Anne Anderson's time.

Which is not to say she is maudlin. On the contrary, when she is not talking about Jimmy's illness or the cluster, her eyes take a lively pleasure in life. Well-liked and surrounded by dedicated friends who feed on her good sense of humor, to the extent that it is possible for a mother to move on from the death of a child, Anne Anderson has regained her personal equilibrium.

To some extent she has changed. Shy and unassuming about her opinions in the early years of her married life, she began to shed her unwillingness to speak up when Jimmy's treatment began, and she never ceased inquiring about what was likely to happen to him next. She acquired the nerve and ability to look a prominent scientist or politician in the eye and say she simply did not believe there was no scientific way to find an answer in Woburn. And once when she was told that the real proof of the hypothesis that wells G and H had caused the leukemias would be if the cluster happened again, exactly the same way, with exactly the same chemicals, somewhere else, she simply said in a characteristically determined but matter-of-fact way, "Doesn't it seem absurd and cruel that it has to happen to others before we can prove it happened here?"

To a woman who has moved the establishment mountain, seen the establishment of an expert panel in Woburn and the acceptance of the "living laboratory" concept, the prospect of a cleanup of the Woburn waste sites, and the enormous amount that has been learned from the Woburn events, progress in Woburn on some levels can be seen as impressive.

But because she feels that what has happened was only what should have logically happened—"if you care about fixing a problem, you will fix it," she says—Anne Anderson still has outsize expectations of the forces whose attention she finally caught.

There are signs of change to note in the attitude of Woburn city government. The former mayor, Thomas M. Higgins, who declined to be interviewed, said only, "My own wife died of cancer, but I myself don't see any point in writing more about it. We have been trying to get out from under a bad name with this thing. We did the best we could with it, and I think it is time to move on." John Rabbitt, however, was elected mayor in 1983 on a platform that he would be frank with the population on the matter of toxic waste. He made a point of staying in touch with FACE in general, and Anne Anderson in particular, in order to be kept informed about new developments in the study of the cluster.

New information is always food for thought for Roland "Pete" Gamache, thirty-three, who was being treated for leukemia in 1985, an adult whose case could not be included in the childhood leukemia cluster figures but who nevertheless lives in the cluster area and is one of the plaintiffs in the Woburn lawsuit. He and his wife, Kathryn, live a few doors from the Zonas, whose son Michael died of leukemia in 1974. Pete was diagnosed on August 1, 1980, after the news of the cluster and wells first broke. "I had felt right along that the water was involved in the kids' cases; in fact my wife and I had given each other a water cooler for our anniversary before the cluster news came out. . . . We were just so grateful our kids weren't involved."

Kathryn Gamache, who grew up in Woburn, feels that East Woburn, not an elite neighborhood, has always been a stepchild in the eyes of the town government, one which did not, for example, ever have sand in the sandbox at school, nor proper sidewalks or signs to divert and slow down the endless traffic that uses the residential neighborhood as a shortcut in and out of Industri-Plex. She says "I am angry because you think you should be protected from these things and you are not. And you have to fight all the time; you fight every day on every level. When we got Pete's diagnosis, we had to walk through the children's treatment area at the hospital. That's when Pete said, 'I am going to lick this; I am just glad it isn't my kids.'"

Pete, whose wife gave him a round plastic pillbox with seven compartments so he can carry his medication in the breast pocket of his workshirt and still keep each dose separate by day, has tried to put distance between himself and the science of his disease. He has chronic lymphocytic leukemia, but he says, "I don't ask too many questions." Prior to his diagnosis he had given practically no thought to death, but he says, "then this happened to me . . . you start to think crazy little things, like will I live to see my daughter's wedding, will I be around to provide for my kids. You ask your doctor what the life span is for something like this, and you hear five to eight years. That is, ah, confusing to hear all of a sudden, when you've been healthy all your life. I bury those numbers."

Pete presses his fingertips against the table rim and looks at his wife. "You just try to live a normal life," she comments, "and we do. . . . Pete doesn't want people to say 'here comes leukemia' when he enters a room."

The special circumstances of the Woburn events generated a level of publicity focusing on the families involved, particularly Anne Anderson, about which she and the others could feel only ambivalent. On the one hand, conscientious publicity is important, essential, if answers to the toxic waste problem are to be found. On the other hand, talking publicly about private anguish does not come naturally to any of the Woburn families. And there is no pat way to answer on live television "how does it feel to lose your child and to know that contaminated groundwater could have been the cause?"

Despite the experience they have gained, sometimes it is difficult for the Woburn families to shield themselves from reportorial insensitivity. For example, despite the abundant newspaper stories written about Woburn and Jimmy Anderson, Anne Anderson will sometimes get calls from reporters who ask her things like "wasn't there some kid who got sick up on Orange Street? Is he still alive?" In fact, the morning after the Harvard study was released in Woburn in February 1984, Mrs. Gamache got a call from a television reporter who asked if Pete Gamache would be willing to be interviewed. Mrs. Gamache said she would have to wait until her husband came home from work to ask him. The reporter said, "Work? Oh well if he is well enough to go to work then I won't do the interview. I thought he was dying."

Having to reduce life and death to a digestible simplicity for others is part of the emotional aftermath with which those who have been touched by leukemia in Woburn live. It poses another ambivalence: the need to move on from the loss of a child and the wish to cling to memories lest they be lost to death as well. All the Woburn parents, for example, remember the exact date their child was diagnosed and the exact time and date of death. In every family where a child has died, parents have a conscious and unconscious repertoire of things they do to retain the memory of their child.

Anyone who has ever been in a child's bedroom can imagine what thoughts small objects might hold—a pair of smudgy sneakers tossed on their sides into a closet, a pile of toy soldiers, stumps of crayons and crayon sharpeners, posters, favorite clothing, decals of rabbits on dresser drawers, notes, drawings, boxes for games long since played without the instructions—all the playthings and belongings of childhood.

Some of the Woburn parents have tried to give their children's clothes away or box up the toys so they will be out of sight, on the theory that it is important not to dwell on sorrow. And yet they are torn by the knowledge that these objects are the record of who it was who lived, slept, played, did homework, and struggled against a fatal disease.

In the Anderson house, black and gold metal letters still spell "Jim" on Jimmy Anderson's door. Anne Anderson keeps a few of his matchbox cars on her own dashboard all the time, not to make her sadder but, it seems, to respect the things that Jimmy liked. A poem she wrote the night of Jimmy's death is prominently placed on a living room wall next to a picture that shows him smiling, happy, and full of the life that would be common to a boy his age. Five years after her son Robbie's death Donna Robbins had yet to open one drawer of his dresser because she knew it was full of his playthings that she did not yet want to see. She kept every single stuffed toy Robbie had; "how could I throw them away?" she asked, "they all had names."

Donna Robbins graduated from nursing school in 1985 and began working in a hospital close to Woburn, while continuing to raise her remaining son, Kevin, then aged ten. Mindful that it would be easy to become overprotective of the brother of a child who died, she watched from her kitchen as Kevin went off to play with a friend and said, "it will be a wonder if I ever let him grow up. I've gotten so paranoid about something happening to him."

On the door of the bedroom Kevin used to share with Robbie, there is a Barnum and Bailey circus poster of the bold lion tamer Gunther Gabel-Williams with tamed lions at his feet. Along the side, where Kevin himself placed it, a simple red and white bumper sticker reads, "Help Fight Leukemia." Kevin talks about his brother frequently, sometimes remembering Robbie's birthday and forgetting his own.

Aftermath did not spare Bruce Young. Still a theology scholar, he has also crammed his bookcases with medical journals and materials on toxic wastes. He incorporated into his sermons such references as, from the 1976 *Litany of Penance:* "For our waste and pollution of your creation, and our lack of concern for those who come after us, accept our repentance, Lord."

Young's approach to theology has always been that parishioners have a basic faith on which they depend, and his role as their shepherd is to add to the maturity of their beliefs, provided the process of adding does not threaten what is already an important bulwark. "I try never to take away a belief without providing something to hang on to." A mature faith, says Young, is not one that accepts any manner of evil and bad luck as God's will and that "puts on God" all the evil of the world. God's will and man's greed are separate realities to Young. He says, "I have gotten tired of half-truths and untruths and the revelations that companies knowingly dumped and said they had not. Their stonewalling, their endless saying, 'not me, not me,' passing the buck because they know how hard these things can be to prove categorically. Sometimes I think morality is spelled M-O-N-E-Y."

There is an emotional aftermath for Young as well. He counsels parents—a mother who deprecates herself because she wants to picture her son's face but can no longer do so; couples who argue about whose idea it was to buy a house in Woburn. Bruce Young himself was personally close to Jimmy Anderson and Robbie Robbins. In fact, he says that one of his greatest contributions to the Woburn events was that he was able to "help some kids get through death," lowering his eyes as he remembers throwing firecrackers with Robbie Robbins against the hospital floor.

Among some people of Woburn there is a lingering cynicism about the city's ability to control its destiny.

Traffic problems grow worse all the time, due to increasing development at the Industri-Plex park and a shortage of roads to divert traffic away from residential neighborhoods. At rush hours, driving in Woburn can be like attempting to force syrup through a straw. Some intersections are outright dangerous. At one there is a warning sign that says, "Bad Intersection Ahead." It would be what some have called a "Woburn solution" to put up the sign and never fix the intersection.

The leaders of Woburn and the community at large will eventually have to face decisions about the future of Woburn's water supply. Since the closure of wells G and H, Woburn has been connected to the Metropolitan District Commission (MDC) water supply, the regional agency that sells water from the Quabbin Reservoir to Woburn and other communities. Woburn had signed a contract with the MDC to obtain water in 1972 and had a piping connection to the system in place in 1974. But because of competing demands on the MDC from other towns, a fire at a main MDC pumping station, and the city's wish to save money by continuing to treat G and H wells for iron and manganese, the MDC water did not actually flow into Woburn until May 23, 1979, the very day after wells G and H were shut down, and the city could no longer avoid depending on the more expensive MDC water.

Though G and H wells are generally described as having been supplementary sources for the town, in fact Woburn was counting on them for an average of 2 million gallons a day in May 1979, or just under half the city's total annual water use at the time.

In 1985 MDC water accounted for about one third of

the city's water use, with the balance coming from groundwater in the Horn Pond area, where the city maintains six wells. According to Robert W. Simonds, public works commissioner in Woburn, the city had been relatively lucky in that its water demand remained relatively constant since 1970, mainly because, despite increased residential use of water, several large industrial users of water left the Woburn area and thereby ceased making heavy demands on the water system.

Given the MDC connection and the Horn Pond wells (which, as of spring 1985, remained free of chemical contamination according to annual tests conducted by the state environmental agency, the DEQE), Simonds believed the city could meet its water demands comfortably into the foreseeable future, given no marked increase in water demand. However, the city did plan to put another well into the Horn Pond area if tests showed the aquifer could sustain more demand. Overpumping, however, could present a critical problem for the town because an overpumped aquifer means that demand for water is sucking away the aquifer's natural ability to recharge itself, and eventually there is no more water to pump. If the situation worsens, land can actually pucker and create the infamous "sinkholes" of Florida where overdevelopment of housing on thin aquifers created conditions in which houses slid into holes in the earth.

The Horn Pond aquifer could be in for other trouble too. Sewage overflow from Burlington, a community just to the west of Woburn, seeps into the aquifer and finds its way to Woburn. According to Simonds, "probably the greatest danger to our Horn Pond water supply is that sewage outflow."

Simonds, of the generation that worried more about bacteria than organic chemicals, must also keep in mind the Merrimac River, which flows south through Burlington and Lowell to Woburn and which is also a source for the Horn Pond aquifer. Burlington became the site of new "high tech" industries, and according to Simonds, "We know the Merrimac used to be perfectly clean until it hit Lowell. I don't know what is going to happen to Burlington in future years. I don't know what they are discharging up there, but if some of those companies discharge into the groundwater, we are in trouble. But it depends on how fast these things travel."

Also, Simonds called the industries in Woburn "clean" from the point of view of water use; that is, they were not big users of water as were the tanneries and chemical companies that have now for the most part left Woburn. But should a large water user wish to locate in the Woburn area, the town would be somewhat hard pressed to provide great new quantities of water without widely expanding its MDC contract.

Another option, of course, would be to reopen wells G and H. While the mayor of Woburn, John Rabbitt, said the wells would never be opened while he was mayor, presumably another mayor could reverse the decision, particularly if it could be urged that the well G and H water could be treated to remove the chemical contamination. In fact, the former mayor of Woburn applied for a grant from the state of Massachusetts in 1983 for $708,000 to clean up wells G and H. The grant was approved, but the money was not allocated.

The idea that similarly contaminated wells could be rehabilitated was certainly in the wind. The nearby community of Acton, which lost 40% of its groundwater supplies to chemical contamination, did install on a pilot basis an activated charcoal filtration system described as being capable of removing solvents such as TCE in the concentrations found in the Woburn groundwater. The Acton treatment plant cost $200,000 to install, of which half was contributed by the W. R. Grace Company, whose dumping practices contaminated the aquifer. Grace also contributed about $9,000 per month to maintain the plant. The $3 million suit against Grace filed by the city of Acton was still pending in federal court as of spring 1985.

The Acton plant was described in an engineering publication as a "model for communities facing similar problems. Until now, financial considerations usually prompted municipalities to seek alternative water sources instead of treating contaminated existing supplies. Acton's experience has demonstrated that treating water contaminated by volatile organics is an economical and viable procedure."

The combination of sharp rise in water demand in Woburn and the availability of technology could push a city administration so inclined toward a cleanup of G and H wells, since the Aberjona aquifer is a source of plentiful water, albeit industrially contaminated and of poor natural quality.

When Anne Anderson heard that Mayor Higgins had requested cleanup funds for wells G and H, she wrote a letter to the *Woburn Daily Times* that said in part, "the news that our present administration is seeking to draw water from a seriously contaminated aquifer seems to say nothing has been learned from the mistakes of the past. I am confident the residents of Woburn are interested in quality water not just quantity."

FACE, of course, opposed any plan to rehabilitate G and H wells and began its own investigation of the water quality at Horn Pond itself. Burlington sewage overflow can, when it rains heavily, discharge right into the pond, and there were a number of tanneries, degreasing plants, illegal landfills, and street runoff pumps in and around the pond. It is also not absolutely clear whether the Aberjona aquifer and the Horn Pond aquifer are completely separate or somehow joined by city drainage systems.

Little attempt had been made by mid-1985 to investigate the extent of wastes buried in the Horn Pond vicinity, and though the city of Woburn knew that sewage outflow did hit the pond every year for some periods, it continued to permit boating and fishing in the pond because its regular bacteria tests showed no worrisome contamination. While FACE continued to argue that the quality of the pond could not help but affect the quality of the aquifer, the Woburn Public Works Department countered that the pond helped "maintain" the aquifer but did not feed it.

Water, for obvious reasons, has replaced the Woburn odor as the talk of the town. And there is now widespread public awareness that the quality of Woburn water is not to be taken for granted. In the lobby of city hall a large MDC poster says, "Water—Our Most Precious Resource," and the conservation commission of the city printed a brochure called "Woburn's Water Supply," which provides basic information about where the water comes from and assures the community Woburn water is safe.

Water too has taken on special significance in the households of the families in the leukemia cluster. Most of them have installed activated carbon filters on their home faucets, despite assurances that the water that comes from MDC is not contaminated. Donna Robbins gave her mother a water filter for her birthday.

Inevitably, in a case like Woburn's where the prospect that ironclad irrefutable proof of a cause-and-effect link will be found is unlikely, a question can be asked about how far investigators can go. Administrators, officials, and scientists who have no direct personal involvement in the matter have the responsibility of deciding when the point has come to close the file. In many cluster cases these decisions are reached on an ad hoc basis. In Woburn the CDC expert panel convened in the spring of 1985 attempted to set some objective criteria for what could otherwise be a subjective process.

The panel recommended that should no additional case of leukemia occur between 1985 and 1989, "the level of monitoring with respect to childhood leukemia be reduced from 'exceptional' to routine," meaning that the detailed following and listing of leukemia cases need not continue, other than through the regular channels of the cancer registry. The "exceptional" methods could also be dropped if the rate of leukemia fell to normal in the years 1990 to 1994.

If there is one child diagnosed with leukemia between 1985 and 1989 in the area of Woburn previously served by wells G and H, and the child was conceived after the wells were closed, then "the hypothesis that the G-H wells are the source of childhood leukemia in Woburn should be considered of doubtful validity." In such a case the panel recommended more data be collected on environmental exposures and "life-style" factors throughout Woburn.

If, on the other hand, there should be a leukemia case in the areas not served by wells G and H, the panel said "we cannot, in this case, reject the "G-H hypothesis. An important contributory factor may be water of the 'G-H type' which does not come directly from the G-H wells; i.e., the contaminants of the G-H wells may be moving into other wells. Therefore, an exploratory study could be done, using the Harvard study as a starting point, for designing and rapidly implementing data collection and analysis."

If in the ultimate case that the leukemia incidence continue at the "present" or an "increased level" regardless of location, what the panel called "clear continuation of the cluster," or three cases in a two-year period, then the situation calls for a "renewed and vigorous effort to identify a cause," a kind of epidemiological crash effort.

The panel also suggested that "the Health Department prepare protocols and sampling frames in the near future in order that a tentative survey could be accomplished in a timely fashion should it be necessary." In other words, the panel put responsible officials on notice that they should be working now on how to take the cluster investigation further, should that be necessary.

It was the first time in the history of the study of leukemia clusters that a cluster, once investigated, was the subject of a deeper, multidisciplinary probe that yielded a set of decision-making criteria for the future and that anticipated the problem of arriving at the future having never done the basic research that would make the necessary investigation possible.

The "renewed and vigorous effort to identify a cause," should it be undertaken, would begin no sooner than thirteen years after Jimmy Anderson's diagnosis and four years after his death. And that is the best science is able to do.

Often Anne Anderson is asked if she is angry. It seems an empty question in her case. Mostly she has expressed her anger in the only channels through which it can course and yield a range of positive results—law, science, and public policy. And she is unwilling to accept that the only system possible is one that cannot, for example, determine the significance of the fact that an East Woburn woman, aged twenty-six, who lived her entire life next door to the Toomey house, where Patrick Toomey who died of leukemia in 1981 had lived, was diagnosed in the spring of 1985 with Hodgkin's disease. This disease, a malignancy that affects the lymph nodes which produce white blood cells, has a longer latency than leukemia, and the woman also was exposed to G and H wells for as long as they were pumping.

That this case of Hodgkin's disease may be related to the leukemia cluster is a situation not even the health monitoring systems recommended by the CDC expert panel would be able to detect. It is therefore extremely difficult for Anne Anderson to be resigned to the reality that, were there to be another cluster in Woburn, it would still take the initiative of citizens to find it first.

Chuck Anderson, who does get mad when he thinks of what has happened and all it has meant to his family, said about what fuels his mother: "I guess the Harvard study was like her revenge. Sometimes I would like to take revenge too. But she did it because she felt she had a moral obligation." He added with the low-voiced pride of a young man who loves his mother very much, "she is all right."

For her part, Anne Anderson does not plan her life very far ahead. While she is mindful that it is important to move on from the events of the past and let them take their course without her, erasing clean is neither possible nor desirable, from her point of view. As she says, "it does not happen cleanly when a child dies. There are years of days of being with that child every moment, of watching the struggle for life being lost, and wondering even years later why it was allowed to happen."

Mostly, she takes life a day at a time because that is the routine that was ingrained when Jimmy was alive. If she projects at all into the future, it is to wonder when all that she has been through to prove an instinct will not have to be endured by someone else. "Finding out what happened in Woburn is the least we can do for children who struggled the way our children did."

She still finds it troubling that childhood leukemia cases can be "disputed," and so to accommodate the registry administrative technicalities of what is and what is not a Woburn "case," she added green pushpins to the map of the Woburn leukemia cluster. As of spring 1985 there were twelve blue for children who died, eight red for children who had been diagnosed with leukemia, and six green for cases FACE assigns to Woburn but the Massachusetts Cancer Registry does not.

"We can remove some of the pins, or change their colors, but it does not remove or change what they stand for," Anne Anderson says. Although she is proud of having helped establish the registry and is aware that it represents great, if imperfect, progress, she has a special reason for knowing it is important.

Prior to the registry, cancer data in Massachusetts were based on information taken from death certificates, which may not always mention cancer as the primary or even secondary cause of death. In the case of Jimmy Anderson, his death certificate reads "pulmonary hemorrhage" as primary cause and "aplastic anemia" as secondary cause. His father, Charles Anderson, who ultimately settled in Canada, said, "it was only when I saw Jimmy's death certificate, only when I looked at the words on the paper, that I realized the full significance of what Anne had been trying to establish all those years." This means that if someone other than Anne Anderson had been trying to quantify leukemia cases in Woburn, Jimmy Anderson would never have been counted.

Ironies in Woburn are sometimes no further away than the telephone. Though the telephone number prefixes in Woburn do not have much geographical meaning, they all, as was true for every telephone in the country, were originally conceived as words. The phones in Bruce Young's office and Anne Anderson's home put them face to face with a short expression of history. The prefixes on their phones, still embossed on Young's, were converted from the old Woburn exchange that used to be known as WE-lls.

Index

401